D1710691

Awake! Aware! Alive!

Exercises for a vital body

Photographs by Steve Hiett
Designed by Adrianne LeMan
Drawings by Diane Nelson

Awake! Aware! Alive!

Exercises for a vital body

by Lydia Bach

 Random House   New York

Among the many who have been helpful in
putting this book together, I would particularly
like to thank Hilary Maddux
of Random House and Mary Jo Ostrum.

Library of Congress Catalog Card Number: 73-4229
ISBN: 0-394-48685-4

Manufactured in the United States of America
9 8 7 6 5 4 3 2
First Edition

for Lotte Berk
with admiration and
without whom this
book would never exist

Author's note

Pregnant women: Most women may do all of the exercises in the warm-up section every day of their pregnancy.If you have exercised before your pregnancy and consider yourself to be very fit, you may attempt the easiest exercises in the stretch section. (The directions say whether the exercise is difficult or easy). *But* do not attempt any other exercise in the book unless your doctor has seen the exercises and given his approval.

Overweight women: First of all, show your doctor these exercises and get his permission to do them. You may do the warm-ups, stretches, and stomach exercises. But if you are fifteen or more pounds over-weight, do very few exercises in the thigh or sex sections. If there is too much fat on top of the thigh muscles, it's as if you're working out with weights on your legs, and you'll overdevelop your thighs ! Concentrate on stretching out your body and working on your stomach muscles until you're not more than ten pounds overweight. Then you may include more exercises, but keep dieting.

Awake! Aware! Alive!

Exercises for a vital body

Introduction

Life should be lived enthusiastically and energetically. Every woman can and should have a body that adds to the zest of her living.

Once you slow down you begin to feel older and everything seems more trouble. Regular exercises give your body the strength, energy, and health of a young body. Even after 40 you can continue to have a youthful zest with the help of carefully planned exercises that are neither time-consuming nor back-breaking. Exercises should never be looked upon as a chore, but rather as part of the pattern of a woman's daily life, and one that gives pleasure and vitality, instead of pain and a feeling of "wasted time." Anything that makes a woman feel beautiful within herself is well worth the time spent. Beautiful as referred to here, is not glamour—it is health, confidence, vitality, and the knowledge that "I feel good about my-self." There is something very exciting and intriguing about a mature woman who has vitality and an increased capacity for living.

I met that very special kind of woman—Lotte Berk—four years ago in Europe. For fourteen years she has been teaching a unique method of exercise which is as precise as a science and contains the most important body movements for a truly strong and healthy body. Some of the most vital women in the world have exercised with Lotte Berk's method, trying to keep their energy and bodies at their peak: Princess Lee Radziwell, Eve Arden, Britt Eklund, Edna O'Brien, Joan Collins, Lady Harlech, Tuesday Weld, Lee Remick, and many others.

After training and studying for a year under Lotte Berk in London, I set out, with diploma in hand, to share with other women this exclusive and valuable method of body conditioning. I started by opening a studio in New York City and called it the Lotte Berk Method. It became so successful that the obvious next step was to make the exercises available to those who could not *come* to the studio; and so, this book.

The exercises in these pages are a combination of the most effective, healthful body move-ments of the method. They include elements of many disciplines including modern ballet, Hatha yoga, orthopedic exercises and the pelvic movements of sex. As such, they are a dynamic combination of physical movements, both pleasurable and functional. This selec-tivity makes for a system of concentrated movements which give miraculously fast results if done conscientiously and regularly. It is not a system designed to slim and trim you down to that "perfect figure," but instead, a system designed to make each woman get the most out of the body she already possesses: a system designed to tone muscles, stretch muscles, and redistribute weight to where it belongs.

Most American women feel exhausted much of the time. Although it is easier to think that this condition is the result of over-exertion and the quickened pace of daily life, exhaustion is often nothing more than a body out of tune with itself. Where we used to climb, run, lift, carry and work hard to accomplish the simplest of tasks, we now have every modern con-venience in the world to free us from or help us with such labors. Although this has simplified our lives and provided us with leisure time, it has also done great damage to our bodies. Some of our leisure time must now be spent in putting our bodies back together again.

Every muscle in our body serves a specific function, although many muscles no longer serve the function for which they were originally designed. The result is that those muscles atrophy, lose their tone, and often change position in the body, making for unattractive bulges and flabby excesses. For example, the stomach muscles are supposed to aid our back muscles and are, in fact, inter-connected. Today, the tendency is to isolate the back muscles (because they are easier to use) and give the back the bulk of the weight in lifts and carries. The result is backache, fatigue, tension and ill health, with the additional side effect of a very unattractive stomach bulge. If we carefully exercise the stomach muscles, we can flatten the stomach while relieving the backache. One of the most unique sections of this book deals with just this problem and consists of a series of orthopedic exercises designed for the woman with back problems caused, most often, by weak stomach muscles. Detailed muscle charts are provided at the opening to four sections to show you exactly what muscles are being worked on in the various exercises and how toning one muscle might very well shape the rest of your body.

At first, you might find the exercises tiring. If you start slowly and do not strain, you will find that the exercises are actually giving you energy rather than robbing you of it, and that your endurance is continually increasing. The rewards are unending, because the possibilities for the body are tremendous. Stretching muscles releases tension and relaxes you. Firming muscles gives you confidence in yourself and also will give you, in time, the contours you would like to see. Even your sex life is bound to improve, particularly through the exercises in the last section of the book.

As you will notice, the exercises are divided up into six sections: warm-ups, stretches, thighs, stomach, bottom and sex. Before beginning them you should be sure you are in good health and consult with your doctor to determine if the exercises in this book are safe for you. Some of the exercises are extremely difficult and should be done only after mastery of the easier exercises has been attained. The exercises should be done, where possible, in the order in which they appear, moving from the simpler to the more advanced as you slowly build up your strength, your stretch, and your confidence. The correctness of your positions are so important that you will need a *full-length mirror* to check your position against the photographs accompanying each exercise. Don't cheat on your positions as they are carefully thought out to give you the maximum benefit with the minimum of discomfort.

Now all you need is music ! Think about your record selection. I don't believe in "exercise-type music." Just choose music that makes you feel good—sometimes I like the Brandenburg Concerti or a Brazilian beat such as a bossa nova, or hard rock like the Rolling Stones. Start the music and keep it playing as long as you exercise. You'll get into the full swing of firming and shaping your body without even realizing that you are exercising.

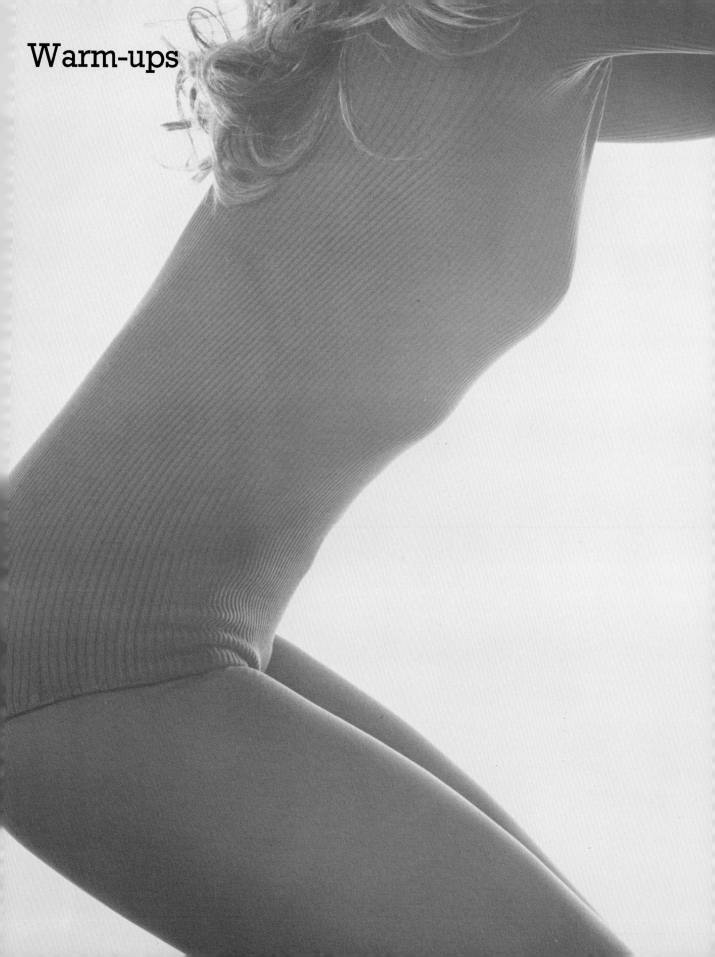

Warm-ups

A   Temporalis
B   Sterno mastoid
C   Trapezius
D   Deltoid
E   Pronator teres
F   Rectus abdominis
G   Tensor fasciae latae
H   Adductor Longus
I   Gracilis
J   Vastus lateralis
K   Extensor digitorum longus
L   Peroneus longus
M   Frontalis
N   Platysma
O   Pectoralis major
P   Biceps brachi
Q   Brachiordialis
R   External oblique
S   Extensor carpi radialis longus
T   Pectineus
U   Sartorius
V   Rectus femoris
W   Vastus medialis
X   Tibialis anterior

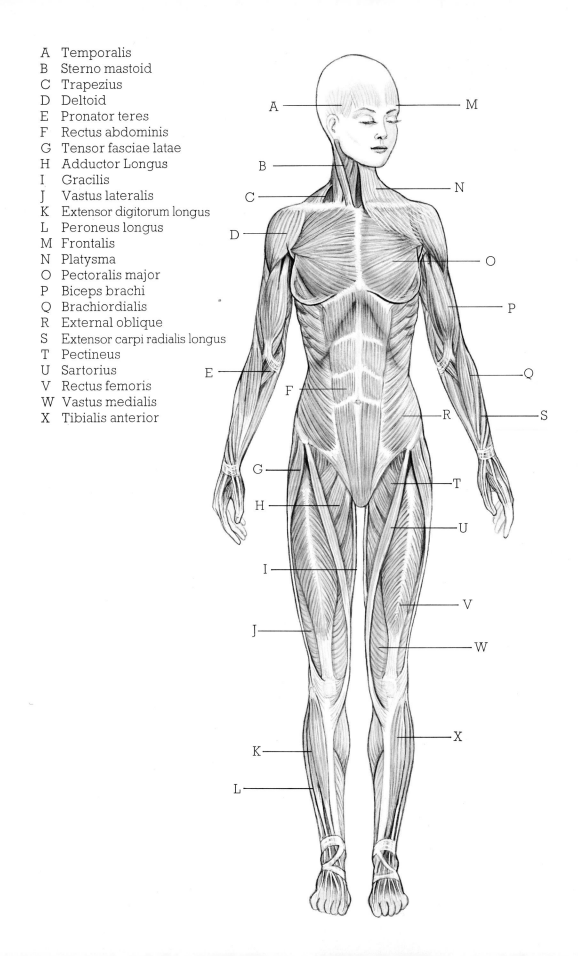

Warm-ups

I feel great when I do all the warm-up exercises every day, and they only take a few minutes. These movements wake up the body because they increase circulation and get a good flow of blood to the tissues and muscles. Good circulation works as a quick "pick-me upper."

After you do all the warm-ups, and your body feels warm and loose, you are ready for specific, concentrated exercises. *Never exercise unprepared or "cold" muscles; you might tear tissues or muscles.* Warming the muscles of your body is like warming the motor of your car. You'll get better performance with maximum effect from the rest of the book when you complete this section.

You may think, I only want to firm my tummy muscles, so I'll skip the warm-ups. Please recognize the danger in only doing isolated movements and follow my advice.

Any healthy woman should be able to do all the warm-ups. The other sections in the book contain graded exercises ranging from beginners to advanced, but all the warm-up exercises are easy enough for everyone.

Throughout the book the pictures are clear and show movement. Before you start, spend time studying the pictures. Next read the directions to clarify the exercise. Lastly, slowly try each step of the exercise *in front of a mirror,* comparing your positions with mine. Don't deviate from the pictures. The correct positioning will give the best results.

Now all you need is music! Think about your record selection. I don't believe in "exercise-type music." Just choose music that makes you feel good—sometimes I like a Brandenburg Concerto or a Brazilian beat such as a bossa nova, or even hard rock like the Rolling Stones. Start the music and keep it playing as long as you exercise. You'll get into the full swing of firming and shaping your body without even realizing that you are exercising.

You should learn your warm-ups after several days. In a few weeks you'll be so accomplished, you'll be able to do all your warm-ups without the book. At any stage of your learning always spend 3 full minutes warming up your body.

Warm-ups—3 minutes.

1   This is the first movement of your warm-ups. Stand with your feet together and stretch to touch the ceiling with your fingertips.

    Bend your knees and swing your arms down toward the floor and behind you. Keep your feet flat on the floor throughout the entire exercise. When you have bent as low as you can and your arms have swung right behind you, *bounce* your knees, swing your arms in a forward motion, and stand straight up again.

    When you have coordinated the movement, this is a very quick swing.

Repeat the movement 7 or 8 times to begin to warm up your entire body.

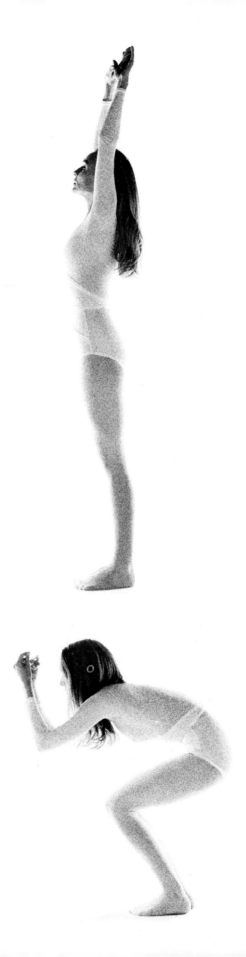

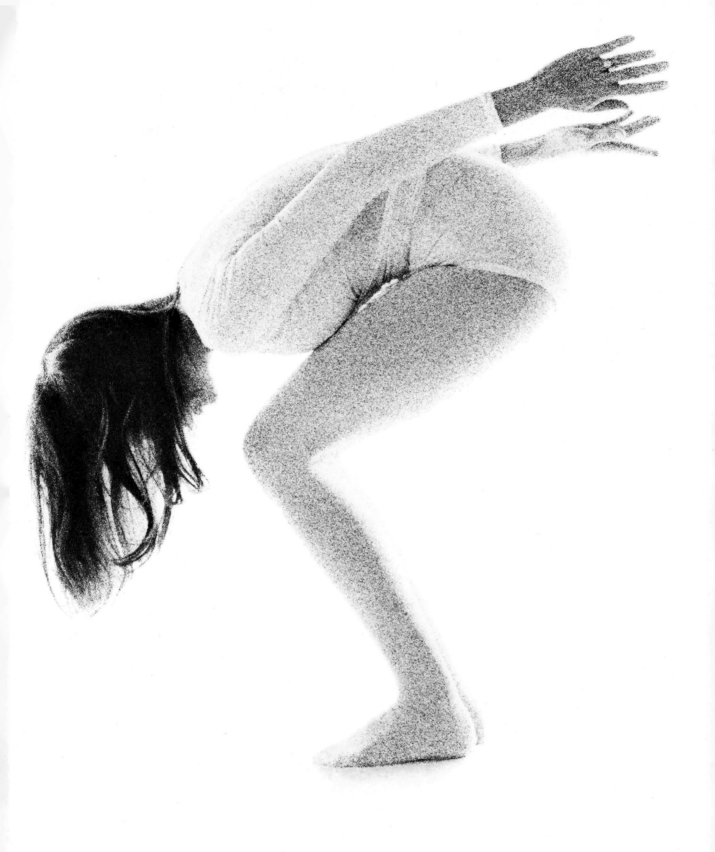

2   Stand with your feet comfortably far apart.
    Stretch your arms above your head toward
    the ceiling. Stretch one arm and then the
    other, as if you were pulling yourself up a
    rope, feeling your entire torso stretch.
    Reach to your fullest height. This exercise
    feels good if you really stretch and stretch.

    Stretch each arm 5 times and hold the stretch
    for 2 seconds.

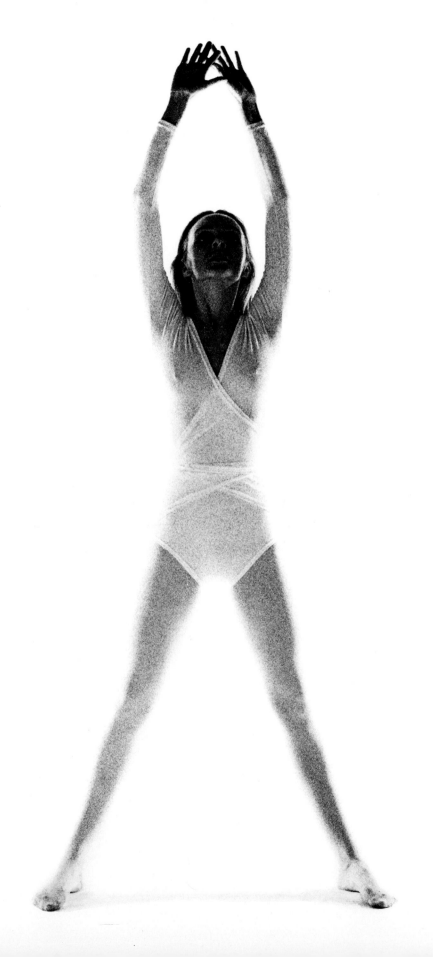

3   This warm-up movement is fantastic for the
    circulation from head to toe as well as
    working on the waist. Stand with your legs
    comfortably far apart with your hands
    resting at your sides. Without bending your
    knees or leaning forward, move rapidly
    from side to side, sliding your hands down
    one side of your leg and up the other side.
    Now watch your stomach profile in a mirror.
    Can you hold your stomach in while you do
    this side-to-side movement ?

    Repeat 10 times.

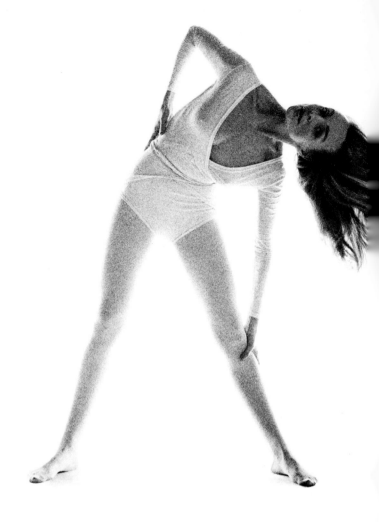

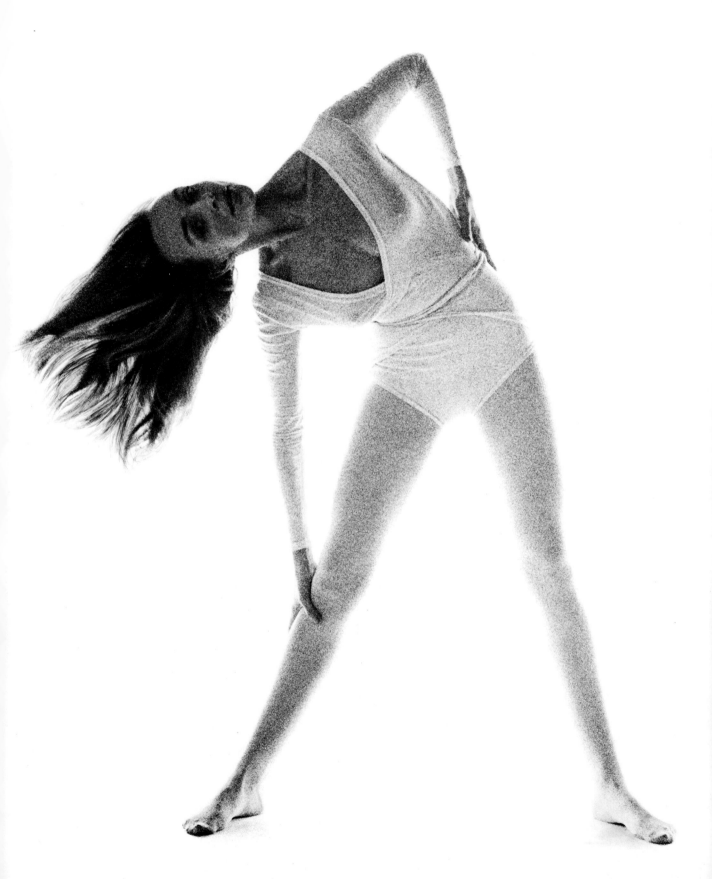

4   Stand with your legs far apart and stretch
    your back parallel to the floor. You should
    feel your spine and the back of your legs
    stretching. Allow your back to curve as you
    bend over and swing your torso and arms
    back and forth several times through your
    legs. Return your body to the first position
    and repeat the swinging motion several
    times.

        Now let your body hang loosely. Grasp
    your inner calves. Be sure your knees are
    straight and pull your torso toward your
    legs. Hold your torso as close as you can
    and count to 5. Don't be discouraged if you
    cannot pull your torso as close to your legs
    as the large picture. Eventually you will get
    closer, but right now work your body
    correctly and stretch only to your capacity.
    The point is to warm up all your muscles,
    not to perform stunts.

    Spend half a minute on these movements.

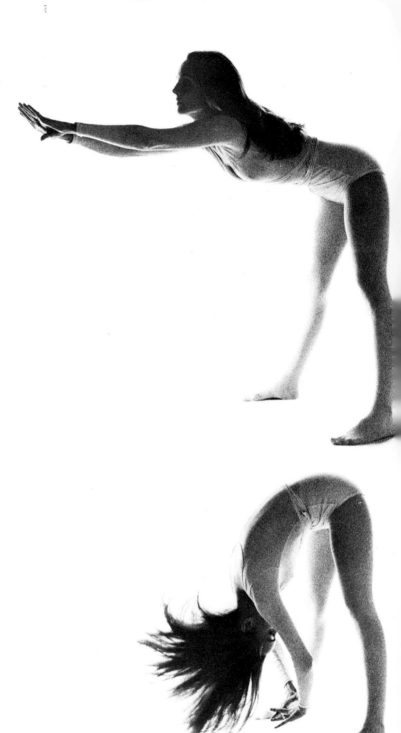

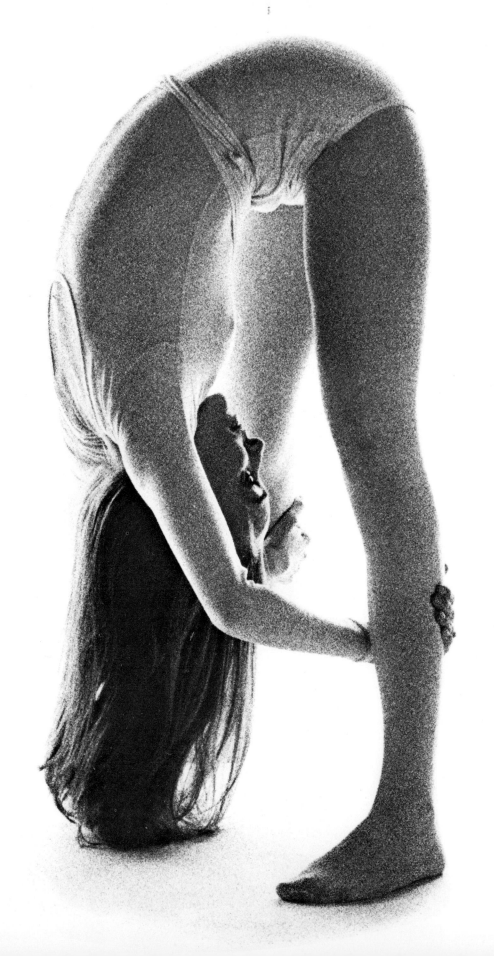

5   Straighten your arms in front of you. Very
quickly cross your hands one over the other
alternately. Note how close the hands are in
the first picture and maintain that closeness.
Keep this small quick movement going until
they've crossed a dozen times or more and
you can feel your arm muscles working.
Relax them. Double the tempo and cross
them 12 times again.

    Now, swing your arms to your side,
shoulder-height if possible. Swing your arms
10 times forward and back, maintaining
shoulder height.

    Next, bend your elbows exactly as illu-
strated in the third picture, fingertips
pointing inward, and try to touch your
elbows behind your back; in this position
push the elbows backward and forward in
small concentrated movements repeating
6 times.

    Lastly, straighten your arms out to the
side and turn your palms forward as in the
large picture and move your stiff arms in a
small circle (the size of a teacup) for half a
minute until you feel a good tightening
of the entire length of your arms.

Spend 1 minute warming your arms and
shoulders.

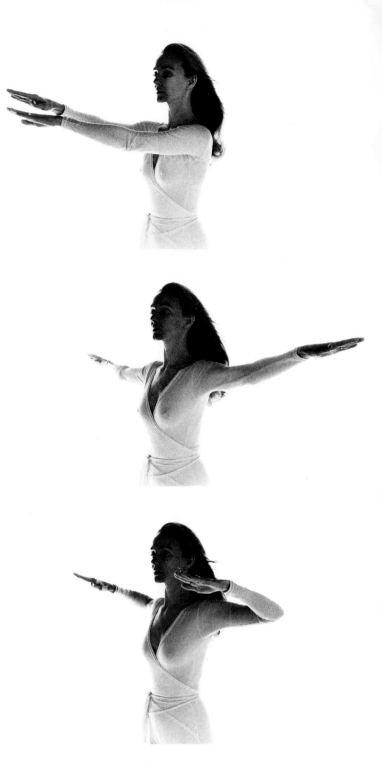

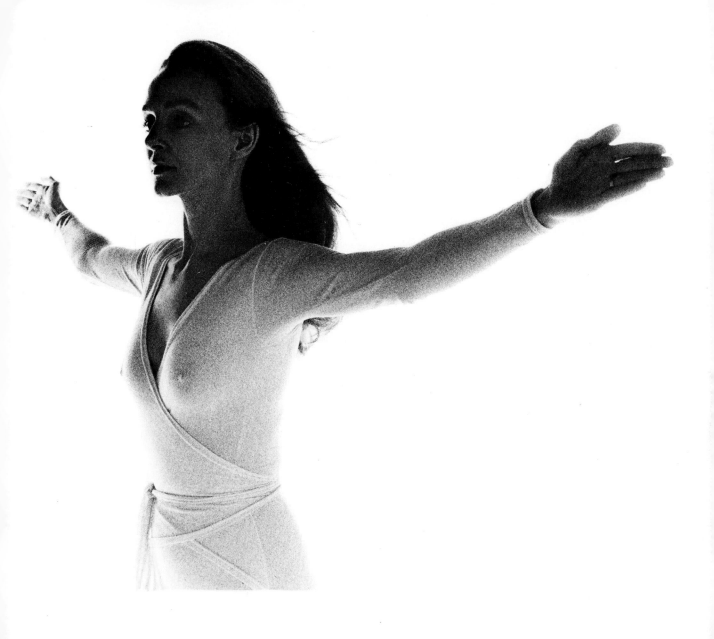

6 Keep your body perfectly still, concentrating
   only on your neck and head. Lift your chin
   as high as possible and look up to your right.
   Now touch your chin to your shoulder,
   slowly dragging your chin across your chest,
   bringing your head around to look upward
   and to your left. Immediately reverse the
   movement. The entire swing should
   resemble a half circle. This makes a beautiful
   movement of the hair if you keep the swing
   constantly in motion. Swing your head in
   time to the music, and you could incorporate
   this head swing with your dance steps.

   Repeat 6 times.

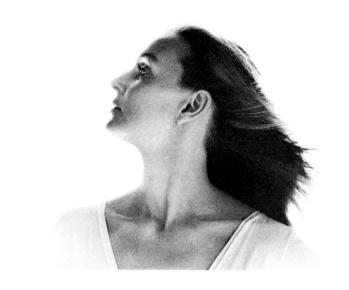

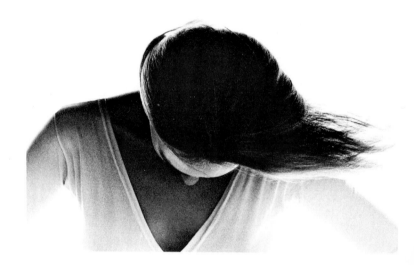

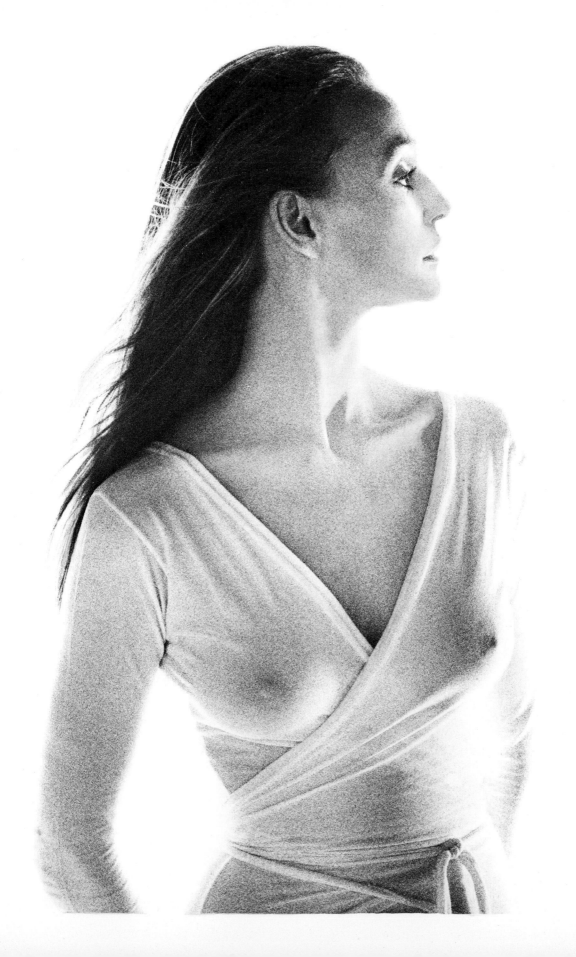

7   Your pectoral muscles "hold up" your
    breasts. Even though it's impossible to en-
    large breasts through exercise alone, you
    can strengthen the *pectoralis minor* to make
    your breasts higher and appear to be larger.
        This is a very famous and successful bust
    exercise. Grasp your wrists tightly and
    pretend you are pushing up sleeves without
    letting your hands slide up your wrists at
    all. This tension should cause a small jump-
    ing movement in the breast area. If you look
    in a mirror while you're doing this, you'll
    see the *pectoralis* tensing and pulling your
    breasts higher.

    Repeat 10 times holding to a count of 3.

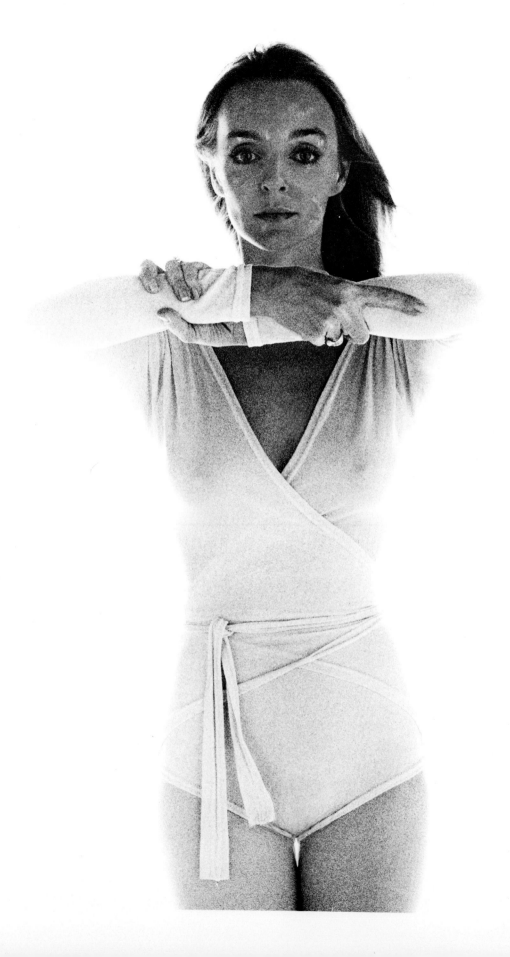

Stretches

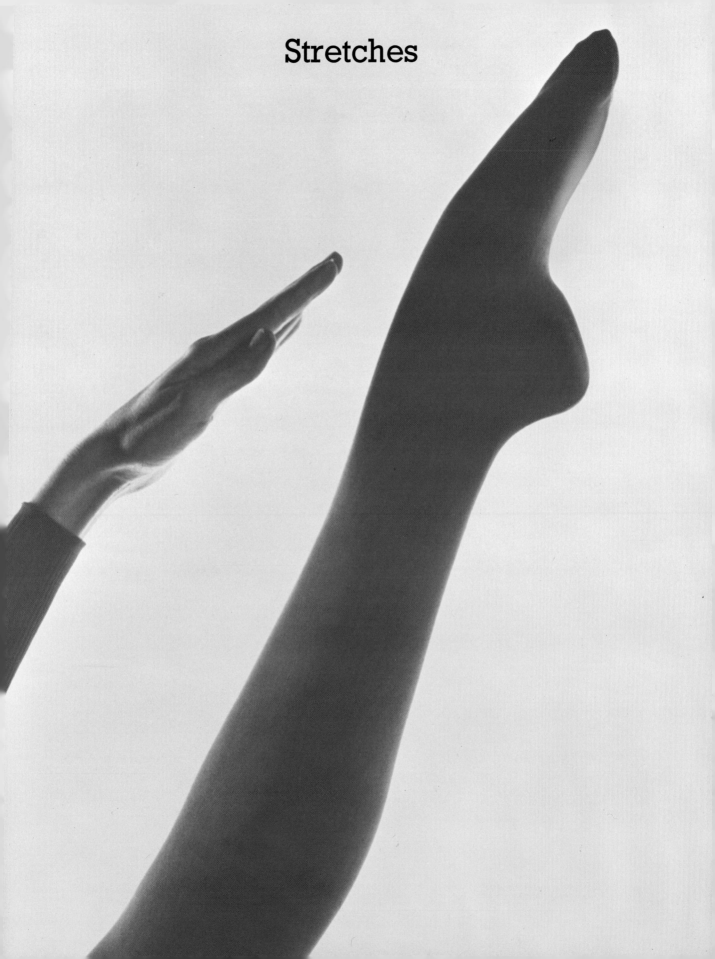

Stretches

A walk that has a bounce of vitality comes from having a limber, loose body. Some people are born with supple bodies, but most of us have to "stretch" very thoroughly to ever become loose. If you are the stiff type, don't be too envious of your more limber friends though, for you'll notice they usually have loose, flaccid muscles. Your stiffness has forced you to use your muscles (not your joints) so you may have a more rigid body but it's also a firmer body.

As we grow older, if we don't exercise our muscles, they will slowly shrink and shorten. It's such a gradual process that we're surprised when we realize at, let's say, age fifty we are no longer the height we were at age twenty. You see, eventually the whole body gets shorter, but this does not have to happen to you. You can stop this shrinking process by stretching a few minutes a day and those few moments can lengthen the muscles and tendons to keep you from shortening.

Many women tell me they actually make themselves grow taller through stretches, but I feel you would have to spend a tremendous amount of time stretching to actually grow, and you would have to reach a very advanced level of stretch.

Stretches make you flexible and graceful. Flexibility is very important in preventing bad accidents that could result in breaks. Imagine a fall if your body is supple. Everything will "give," and you'll go with the fall. More than likely, you'll not break any bones. When an accident occurs and you're rigid, your body doesn't "give"; your bones give, instead, and are fractured or broken.

As you can see, stretches are as important a daily discipline as the warm-ups. But don't mistake stretches for warm-ups. Before you do any stretch, complete all of your warm-ups, or you could tear a tendon.

In the beginning of the chapter I'm doing some easy stretches, but my degree of stretch is advanced. Try to understand the importance of that statement so you won't be discouraged by the pictures. My positions are easy but my legs may be wider apart or my face may be closer to my knees. Position your body exactly as I do in the pictures following every word of the directions carefully, but don't worry about how far you can stretch in the beginning. Stretching takes time and comes slowly, but it does come if you'll try with me. Start right now. Don't allow any interruptions. You should be stretching for the next 3 minutes.

Spend 3 minutes on your stretches.

8   This stretch in yoga terms is called pincers or spinal stretch. It has the twofold advantage of exercising the spine and stretching the back of the legs. Sit on the floor, place your feet and knees close together, hold your ankles firmly, and gently pull your chest down to your knees. Make sure your knees are straight throughout. When you are as low as you can get, bounce your torso slightly to stretch even further.

If you are very supple, try to touch your face to your knees and hold for 10 counts!

If you are very stiff and cannot reach your ankles, hold onto your knees or calves at first. Very gently pull your torso forward.

Go as low as you can, hold for a count of 10.

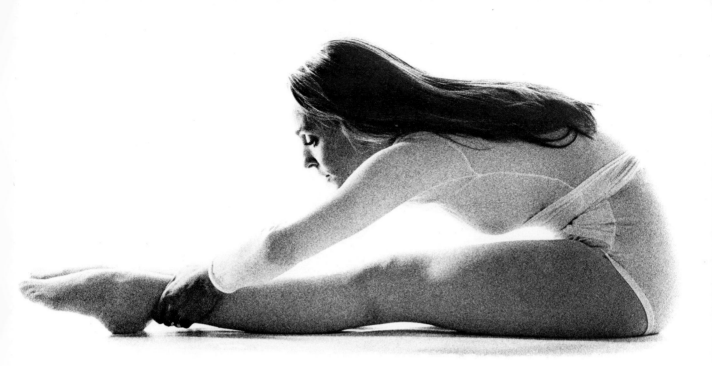

9   Kneel on the floor with knees and feet to-
    gether. Place your hands on the floor be-
    hind you and push the pelvis up as far as
    your thighs will allow. (Feel that stretch?)
    Don't change position, repeat 4 or 5 times
    holding the stretch for 10 seconds. If this
    seems too easy for you, attempt the next
    thigh stretch.

    Repeat 4 times and hold for 10 seconds.

10 **Warning: This is an advanced stretch! If you
    are going to attempt this exercise, follow
    the directions slowly and carefully.**

    Kneel on the floor with knees slightly apart
    and feet together. Sit on your heels and
    place your elbows on the floor behind you.
    Push the pelvis up as far as your thighs will
    allow. Do not force this or any other stretch.
    Your stretch will improve with practice.

    Do this once, but hold for 10 seconds.

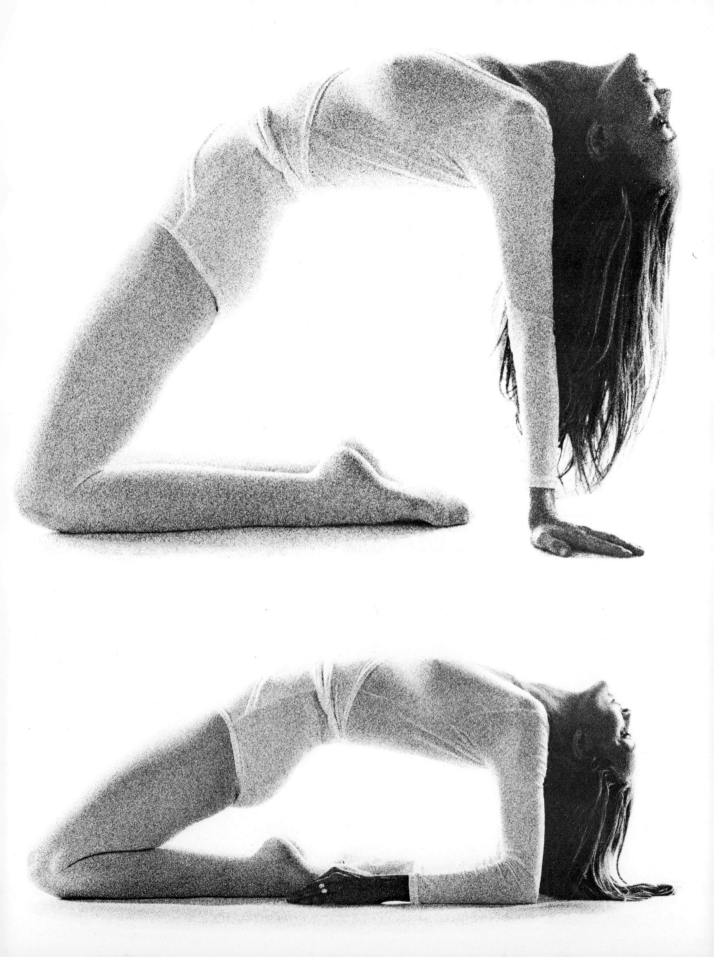

11 Sit in a proper ballet stretch; that is, stretch your legs as wide as they will open, to your *own* capacity. Again don't be discouraged by my stretch. I really don't expect you to be very open for several weeks. Now point your toes, and stretch your arms well above your head. Lean to the left and be sure your arms are in the exact position as in the picture. As you lean directly over your outstretched leg, lower your torso as close to your leg as you can. You should feel a very strong pull along the opposite side of your waist.

Straighten up again and lean over to the other side. Stay with the first two pictures if you are very stiff. With practice you'll be able to advance to the 3rd picture. If you are very "stretched out," try the *advanced* move and turn your upper torso till you are facing your leg, hold onto your ankle, and attempt to touch your face to your knee. Hold for 10 seconds.

Stretch on each side, hold for 10 seconds.

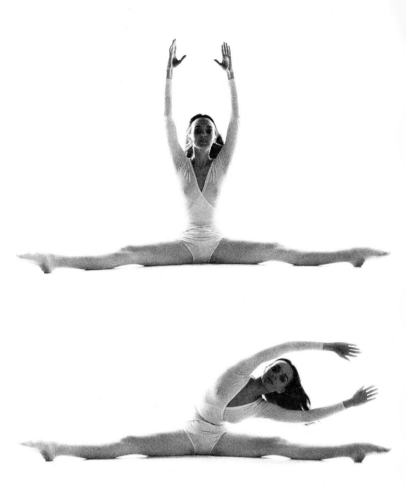

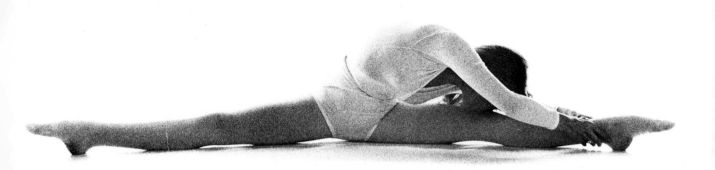

12   **Warning : advanced stretch only.**

In Yoga this position is *halasana :* the plough.
Your neck must be supple to complete this
position. Be very careful and start slowly. Be
totally aware of your spine stretching and
don't force the stretch, Beginners follow the
directions, but keep your legs bent if they
do reach the floor. To start, lie on your back.
Gradually raise the legs, thighs and torso into
a vertical position with the palms supporting
the small of the back. When the vertical
position is reached continue tilting thighs and
legs over your head till your toes touch the
ground, feet apart. Then lay your hands flat
on the floor out to the side.

   Hold to a count of 10. Are your knees
straight? Then relax, reversing the instruc-
tions so you are lying on your back again.

Complete once and hold for 10 seconds.

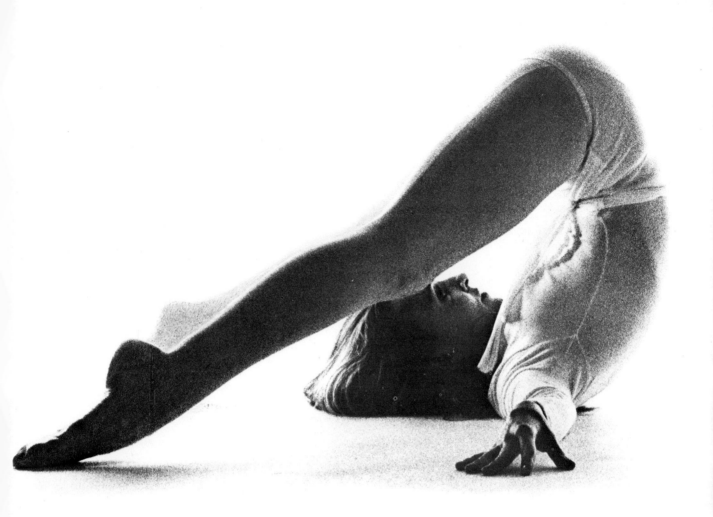

13 Stand with your knees and feet close together, and clasp your hands behind your
back. Raise your arms upward, as you
slowly lower your head toward your knees.
At first, just concentrate on trying to keep
your balance, as you aim for your knees.
Remember to keep the knees straight, even
if you don't get down very far at first. You'll
get better results if you do each step cor-
rectly rather than rapidly trying to reach the
goal.

Lower once as far as you can and hold for
10 seconds.

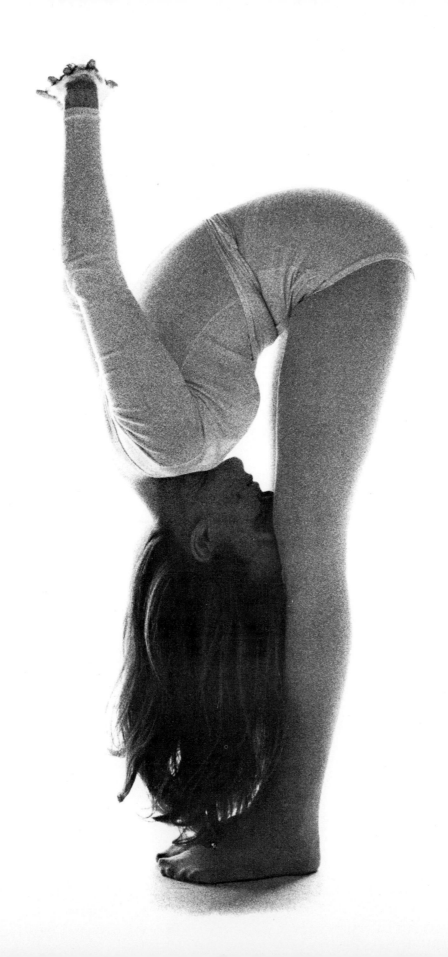

14 Advanced stretch and balance.

This is a stretch-and-balance exercise that
stretches the spine and all the muscles down
the back of your legs. Make sure you have a
lot of space around you. You might fall over
very rapidly and hit any furniture or wall that
may be near you.

Find a comfortable sitting position, knees
and feet together; now bend your knees up
to the chest. Grasp outer heels, slowly
straightening legs up above your head till
they're almost perpendicular to the floor.
If you can balance on your tail bone, try to
touch your head to your knees. If you have
the stretch but not the balance, lean against
a wall and try again. Beginners, try one leg
at a time.

Complete once, hold for 10 seconds.

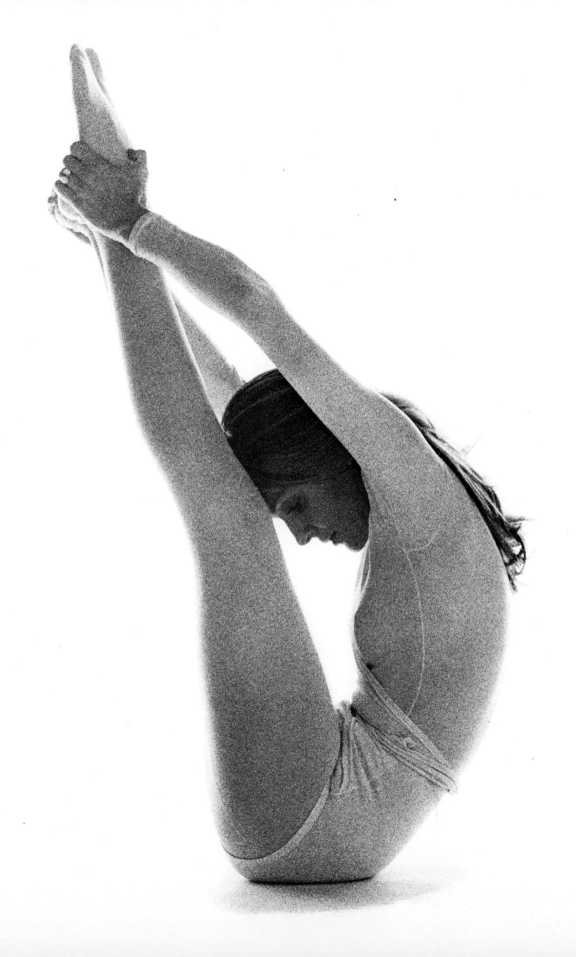

15 Final and most advanced stretch.

In Yoga this position is called the angular pose. It's a combination of balance and stretch as is the previous exercise, but it stretches the inner thighs as well as the spine and back of the legs. You can reach this position with patience and practice, but at first do not expect to be able to stretch and balance to the extent shown in the picture. For now just try the stretch using a wall to lean against. You can move away from the wall when you've perfected the stretch.

Sit with legs slightly apart and lean back against the wall, resting weight on your tail bone.

Bend knees and grasp insteps.

Now straighten legs as wide as you can.

Hold this position for 10 seconds and feel the tremendous stretch along the inner thighs and backs of legs.

When you've developed your stretch and you feel that you have the balance, don't use the wall anymore. Just be careful that you have plenty of room behind you in case you roll backwards quickly and hit something.

Beginners : follow the directions stretching one leg at a time.
Try once and hold for 10 seconds.

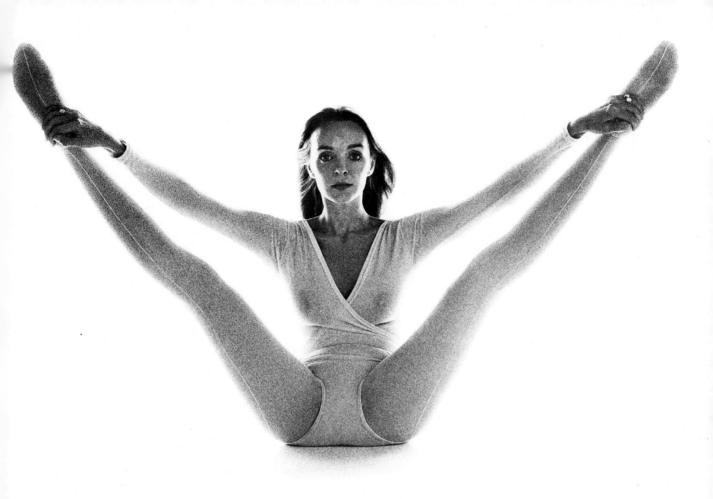

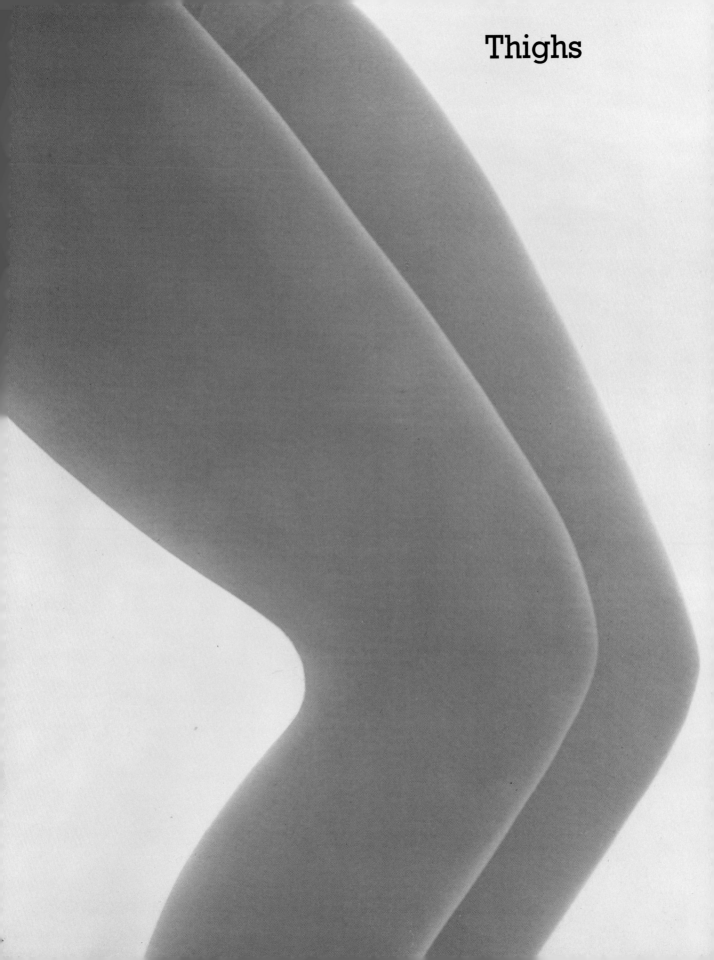

Thighs

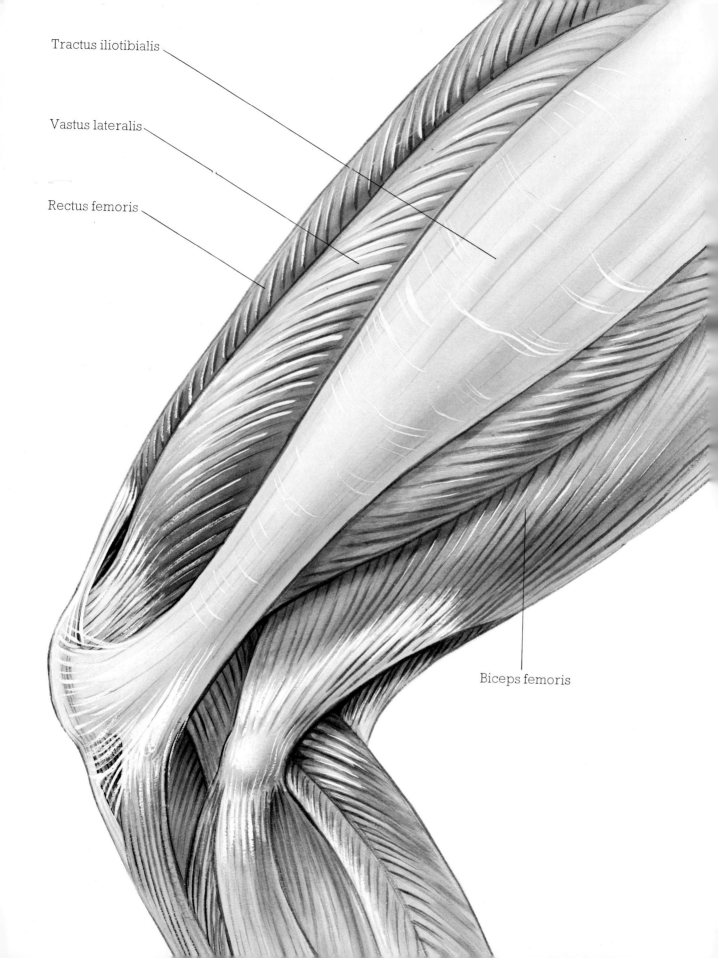

Tractus iliotibialis

Vastus lateralis

Rectus femoris

Biceps femoris

Thighs

Your thighs are the easiest part of your body to firm. Why is that? Look at your muscles in the chart. They are long and large so they are fairly easy to firm with exercise. Probably the worst part of getting thighs firm is the agony you'll go through the first week or so. If you're flabby with small lumps, you'll get sore; if you're firm but unexercised, you'll get sore. There is no way of getting around that initial discomfort and ache.

The stiffness alone should make you realize that you've let yourself get out of shape. Now force yourself to get over this uncomfortable stage, so you'll never be sore or flabby again.

Test yourself in the beginning to see what kind of condition you are in. Try only the first exercise in this section for 10 days but **precisely** as directed. No cheating! Turn the page and examine the exercise. By the directions you'll understand there's a Midway Point that you must learn and **hold**! After 10 days of teaching your body that stress point, start to increase your thigh exercise adding one a week.

One bit of advice. You will be the most uncomfortable the second day after you do the thigh exercises. Please don't quit and wait until the soreness goes away to start again. The fact is that you must continue exercising every day to get past the sore stage. Cold muscles are stiff and uncomfortable; warm muscles get loose and feel better.

Let's look again at the muscle chart so you understand your thigh muscles before you exercise them. Look at your superficial muscles. They run from your hips to your knees. If they get stiff or sore, you're going to feel it more than any other part of your body because you have to use them to **move.** You need those thigh muscles to walk, sit, go down stairs (and when those muscles get sore, you will find it more difficult than going *up* stairs).

Are you wondering why muscles are so flabby and weak if you have to use them to move? Our movements in the twentieth century are very restricted—especially those movements of city people. We rarely walk great distances or run or jump. We just don't use our muscles the way we used to.

Many women ask me if they can reduce their thighs with exercise. The answer depends on how much of the thighs is fat and how much is muscle. Exercise won't get rid of the weight, only less food will. But *proper* thigh exercises can tighten and firm the thigh muscles which will reduce their size. Even overweight women tell me they feel thinner when their bodies are firm. Smooth muscles look better and trimmer than soft, loose flesh.

Let's see how much of your thighs are fat and how much are soft muscle. While standing, raise your leg in front of you as high as possible and hold it high, using your thigh muscle. Press your fingers into the front of your thighs to feel the muscle. Continue to keep your leg raised. Now "pinch" the flesh on top of that front muscle. If you can pinch over 1 inch, you need to lose weight, but if you pinch less than 1 inch your thighs are mostly muscle. If they are flabby when relaxed, you only need to firm them. Flab is soft, unused muscle; it is not fat.

First, study the pictures carefully.

Find a heavy chair or dresser waist-high, and put it in front of a mirror. Grasp it firmly. Stand on the *very tip* of your toes and stretch to your tallest. Hold your shoulders as straight as mine in the pictures.

Slowly bend your knees, but keep your back straight and "keep on your toes." *Note the position of my feet in all the pictures.* Lower your body all the way to your heels and sit on your heels.

From sitting on your heels raise your body with your thigh muscles (not your arms) to the Midway Point, as shown on the opposite page. Hold to a count of 5. Stand up and shake your legs well to de-tense and relax the thigh muscles.

The Midway Point is the level of greatest stress. Your body will try to avoid that level, but the Midway Point is going to get the fastest results. Let's start all over again. Very sternly, watch your body performing for you in the mirror, and try to duplicate the 1st, 2nd and 3rd pictures. If you reach the 3rd picture and have followed strictly all the requirements, hold to a count of 5 and lower slowly with thigh control to your heels. Take a break and look back and forth between the 2nd and 3rd pictures—you will get an idea of the movement : up, *hold* – down, relax – up, *hold,* etc.

Don't be surprised if your legs are a bit shaky at first. That means the muscles are in action again, and they are unsure of themselves. Ease up today, but get back at them tomorrow.

Hold the Midway Point : Beginners : hold to a
slow count of 2 or 3.
Advanced : hold to a
slow count of 15.

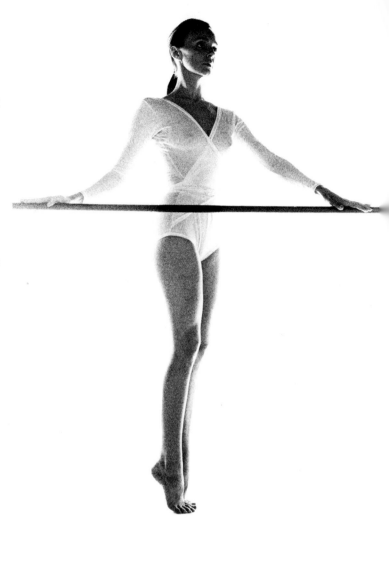

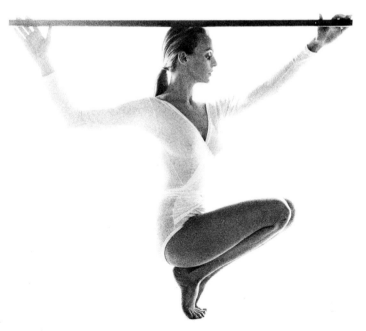

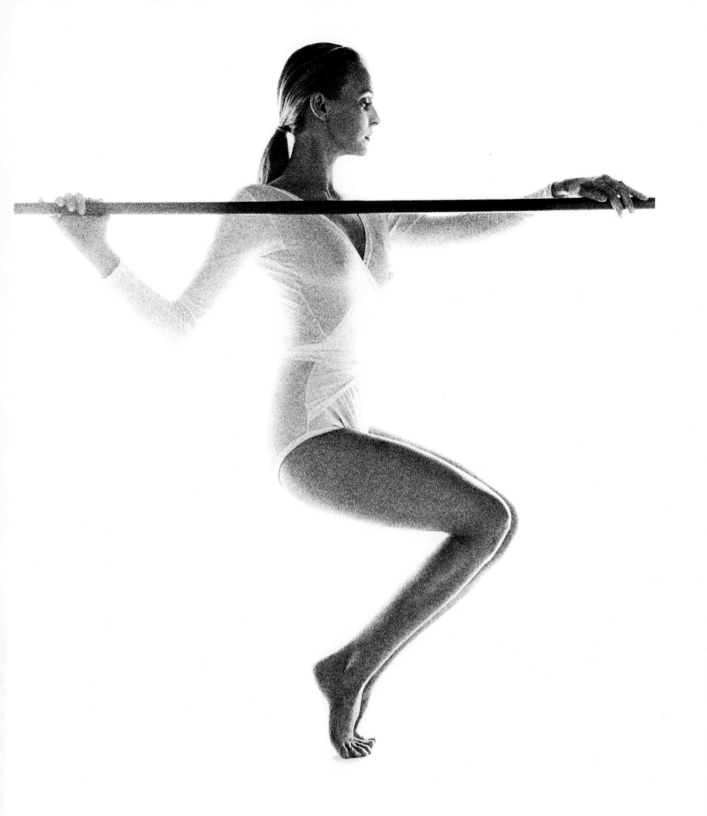

17 Very advanced.

If you are confident of your thigh strength from the previous exercise, you are ready to attempt this movement.

Get the heavy chair in front of the mirror again. Stand up very straight and balance all of your weight on the very tip of your toes, stretching your left foot in front of you. Lift your leg at the height you are able to. (Waist-high is extremely advanced.)

Now bend your right knee and lower your body as low as possible, not losing the height of the left leg. Keep your control and straighten your right leg, attaining your full height again.

Don't relax. Try to repeat the bending and straightening movement of your right leg. Once more for beginners, 5 more for advanced.

Remember—you have two legs. Change legs and repeat the movement.

Bend-straighten 2 or 3 times.

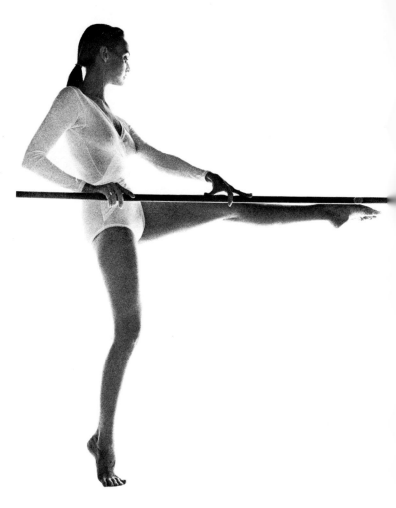

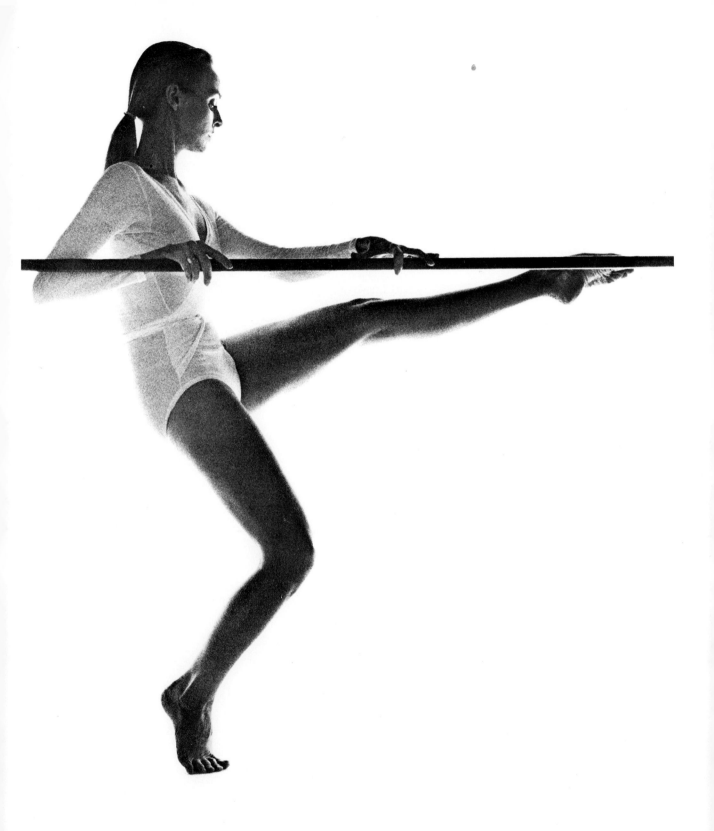

18 Use the back of a *heavy* chair, approximately waist-high and put it in front of a mirror. Grip the chair. With feet together open your knees as wide as possible and slowly sit on your heels, using your thigh muscles to lower you. Don't lean on the chair—use the chair for balance only. As you lower your body, your back must be perfectly straight. Slowly raise your body to that Midway Point and hold this point to a count of 10. (You should have learned it in the first exercise of this section.) Now slowly "work your pelvis," thrusting your hip first to the left, then to the right, and moving from one side to the other until you've lowered your body *with control* to your feet again.

Repeat 3 times.

More advanced variation of the above exercise.

Look rapidly from the first to the second picture. See the up and down movement? Try to duplicate that. Sit on your heels. Raise your body to the position in picture 2 and lower quickly back to position 1. Keep this up-and-down movement going till you've raised and lowered your body 10 times. For variation another day, hold the position of picture 2 and bounce your body in a small concentrated up-and-down movement.

Up-and-down 10 times.

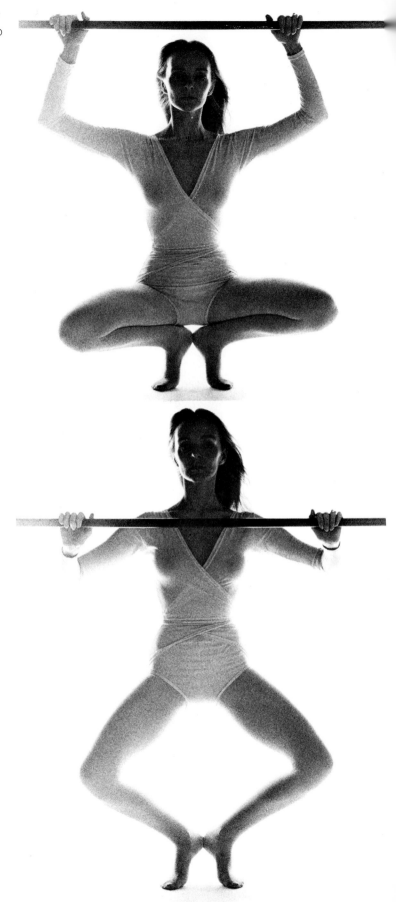

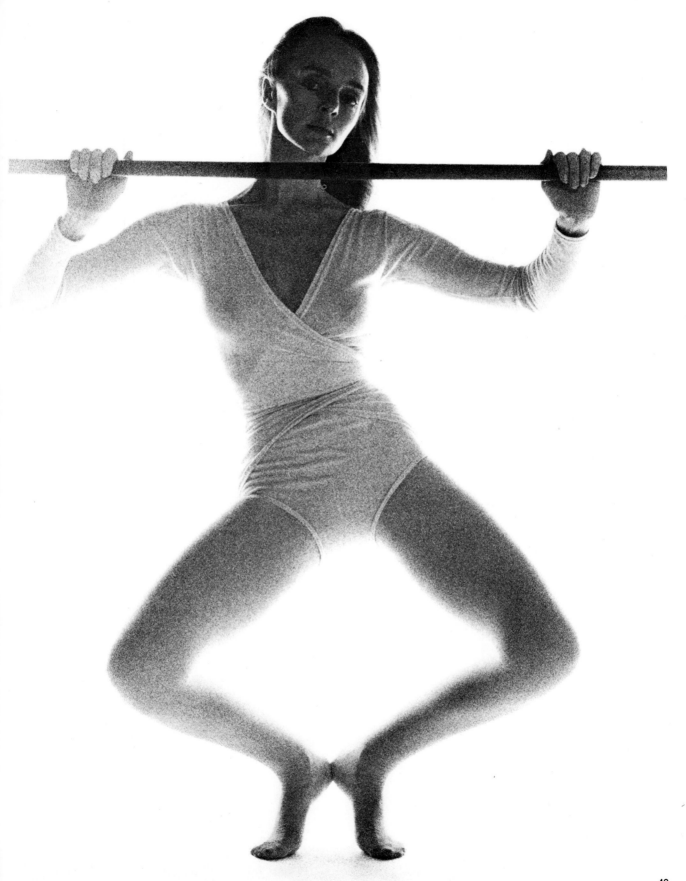

19 Use a waist-high dresser and rest your left
leg on it. Point your toes, stretch your left
leg, and slowly raise it off the ledge. You
should have difficulty at first raising your leg
as high as the picture, so don't be discouraged. It is more important for your back
and both your legs to be straight than for your
left leg to be very high. Watch these points
and try holding your left leg at a lower level.
Change legs and try raising your right leg.

Once you've achieved the basic stance,
try to keep your right leg straight. Place
your left leg on the ledge. Lift the left leg up
as high as you can and bend and straighten
your left knee. **This is an advanced variation
of the exercise for you to work up to.** Change
legs and repeat on your right leg.

Try 4 holds, relaxing your leg on the ledge
in between holds.

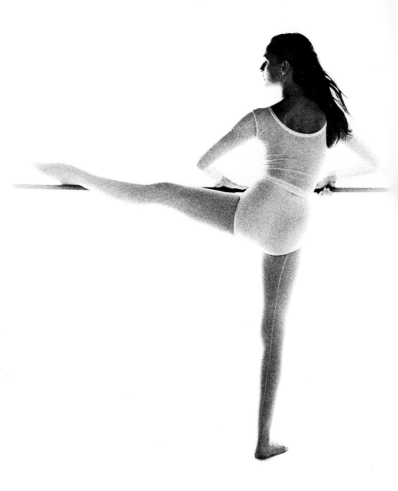

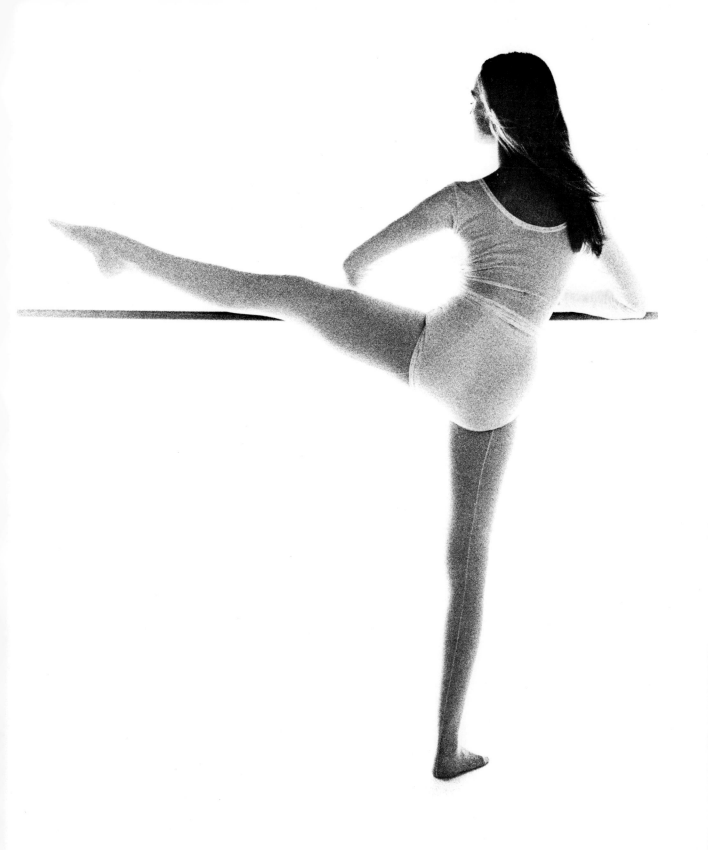

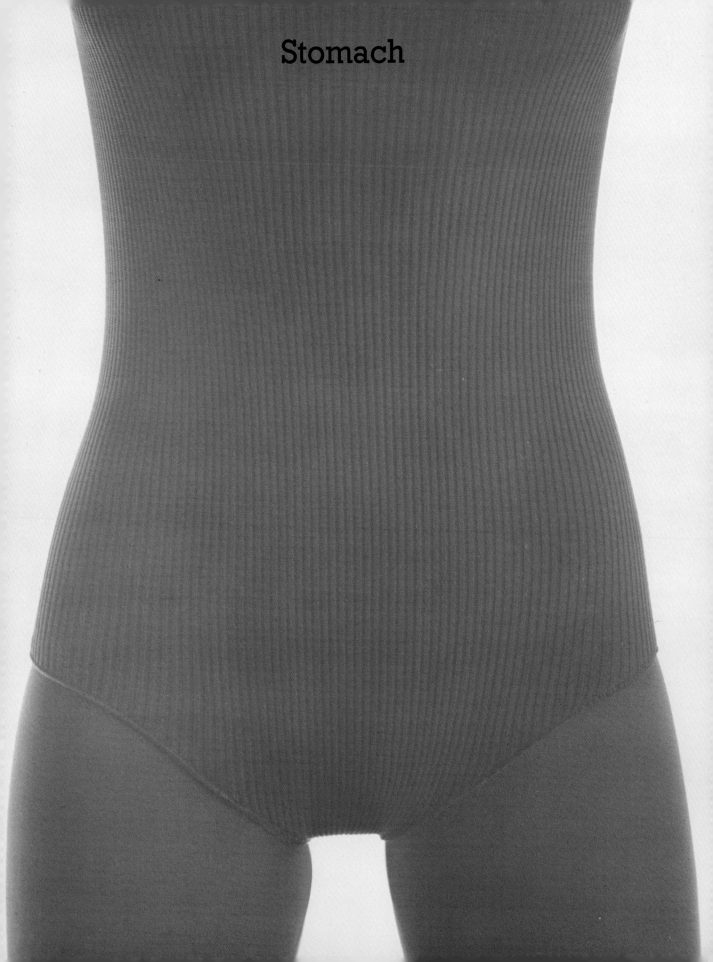

Stomach

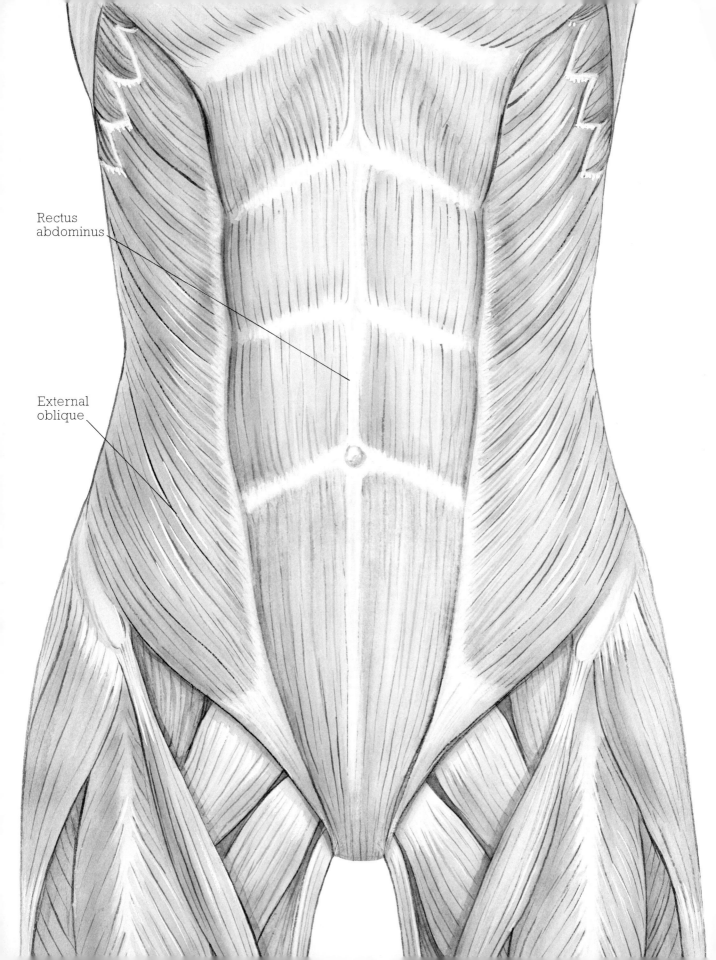

Rectus
abdominus

External
oblique

Stomach

To tighten and firm your stomach muscles,
you'll be learning what I call "firming
tension." It starts below the bust and works
its way to your waist. After a few weeks when
your stomach muscles are much stronger,
the "firming tension" will travel to your
lower abdominal area. The stomach muscles
are so difficult to reach that once you do feel
them, discipline yourself to sustain the
tightening as long as directed. When you
can no longer hold the position, allow your
body to relax completely and breathe deeply.
Unlike the thighs which are shaky and tense
for a few hours after they have been exercised, stomach muscles relax the minute you
stop working them. This is the second reason
you must force yourself to hold or maintain
some of the positions I am going to show you.
While you are holding the position, you
should be able to feel the tension mounting
in your stomach muscles. Remember this is
firming tension and will really flatten your
stomach, so bear with the discomfort and
don't relax until you absolutely have to.
When you do give in, breathe deeply, and
get started again.

**If you feel any discomfort in your lower
back, re-read the exercise—get in front of a
mirror—and watch yourself very carefully.**
You must be doing some part of the exercise
incorrectly. These are orthopedic exercises
for bad backs, so you shouldn't feel any pain
in your lower back.

Now look at the first exercise in this
section to understand the following para-
graph better. During the first few weeks you
may feel two side effects, neither of them
harmful a: slightly stiff upper back, and a stiff
neck. Notice how my back is "rounded" in
the photographs. The stretched feeling
across the shoulder blades comes from this
"rounding of the back" which is done by
pulling on the inner thighs with your hands.
Don't let this feeling worry you. You probably have a fairly stiff *upper* back, and this
will help you to loosen up. The stiff neck is
caused from the neck muscles trying to take
on some of the work load of the lazy
stomach. Let the neck help out at first; it can
only get firm. Later the stomach will get
strong enough to exercise alone.

You must exercise the stomach 6 minutes.

20 This is a very unusual stomach exercise, for it can be immediately effective, as you will feel, if you carefully follow the movements. Get in front of a mirror and watch yourself very closely. *Your body may not be doing what you think it is doing.*

Now examine all the pictures carefully. Note the subtle difference of the position of the back to the floor. The lower the back goes, the more strength is needed by the stomach muscles. The first time you try the exercise you probably won't feel the stomach muscles working very much; but continue to try the positions, studying the directions and pictures. *Very soon* you will be able to feel your stomach tightening.

Sit with a very straight back and place your feet and knees several inches apart. Grasp firmly the inner thighs with your hands. Make sure your elbows are as high and open as the first three pictures.

Pull your inner thighs hard toward you, using them as leverage to round and stretch across your shoulder blades. As you "round your back," start to lower your back toward the floor. You should feel a definite stretch across your *upper back.*

Lower your back slowly until you feel the small of your back touch the floor. Then let go of your hands and stretch them above your head. Hold to a count of 10 then relax by lowering your back to the floor gradually.

Hold to a count of 10.

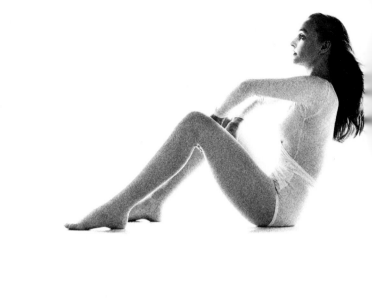

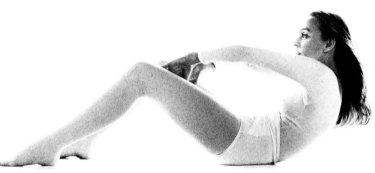

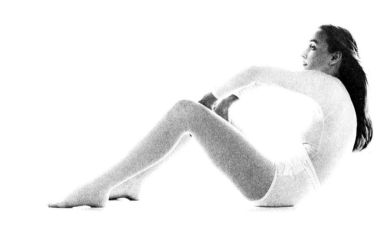

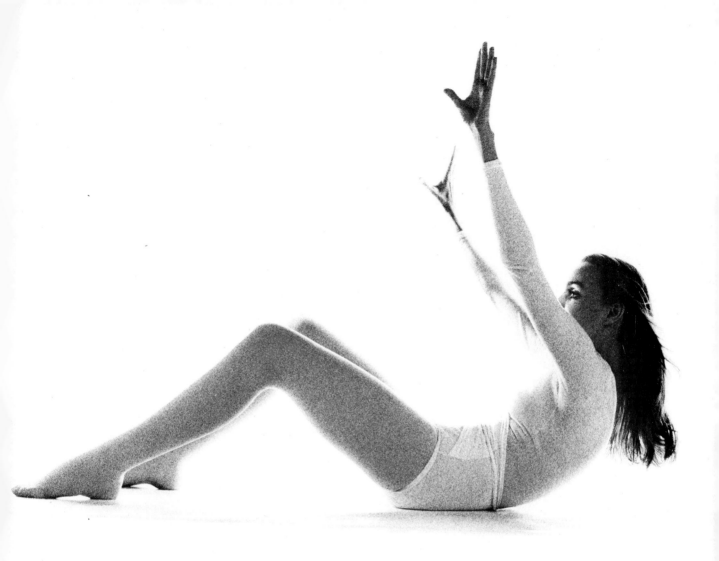

21 Sit on the carpet and bend your right leg, but
    do not let the foot come off the floor. Grasp
    your thigh firmly with both hands and "round
    your shoulders" as explained in the previous
    exercise. Slowly and carefully lower your
    back to the floor. When you feel the small of
    your back touch the floor, let go of your
    hands and reach in front of you without
    altering the position of your back. Count
    slowly to 10. Now change legs and repeat
    entire exercise.

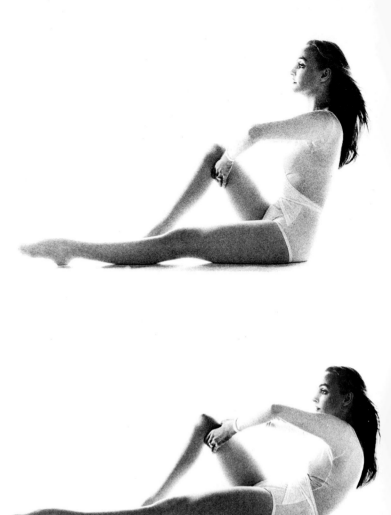

       At first most women position themselves
    fairly well, but when it comes to letting go of
    their hands, the small of the back pulls away
    from the floor and the back straightens out.
    This only means your stomach muscles aren't
    strong enough to hold the back in such a low
    position. It does not mean that you are not
    "working" your stomach muscles. Place
    your hand on your stomach while you're
    doing this exercise and you'll feel the
    stomach muscles tightening ! To work your
    stomach muscles at a less advanced level,
    study the 2nd picture. This will be your
    working level from now until your stomach
    is stronger. Follow all the directions, but let
    go of your hands at the level of the 2nd
    picture, not the 3rd. Don't forget your future
    goal is the last picture. You'll work "down"
    to it with patience.

    Lower back—hold to a count of 10.

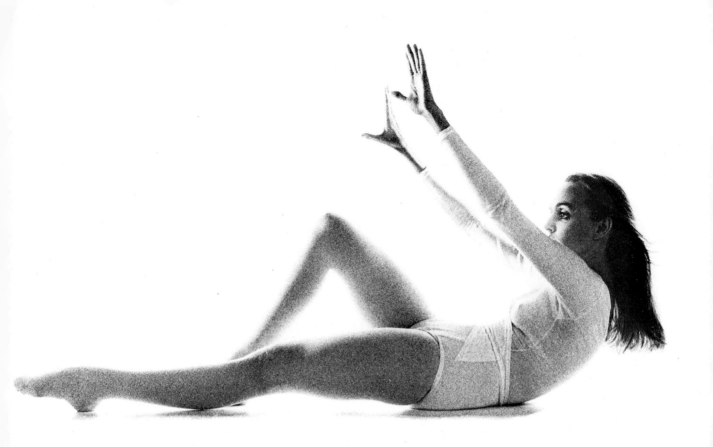

22 Advanced.

When you have mastered the first two exercises of this chapter, you will be ready to add these more advanced arm movements.

Reach the ultimate position of either of the two preceding exercises, keeping the small of your back touching the floor and your shoulders rounded. Imitate the arm positions in the 1st and 2nd pictures; first stretch up high above your head, then cross your arms *behind* your head and actually try to hold your shoulders.

Repeat 4 times without letting the back lose its position.

Look at the arm movement of the 3rd and 4th pictures. You will lower yourself once again to the level you can reach of the preceding exercise and hold that position. First raise the left arm over your head and extend the right arm to your side. Change arms. Once you can hold these positions, try swinging your arms in an arc over your head from one side to the other.

The larger picture is a wide extension of the arms. You should be able to hold this position for 10 seconds with your back in the proper position.

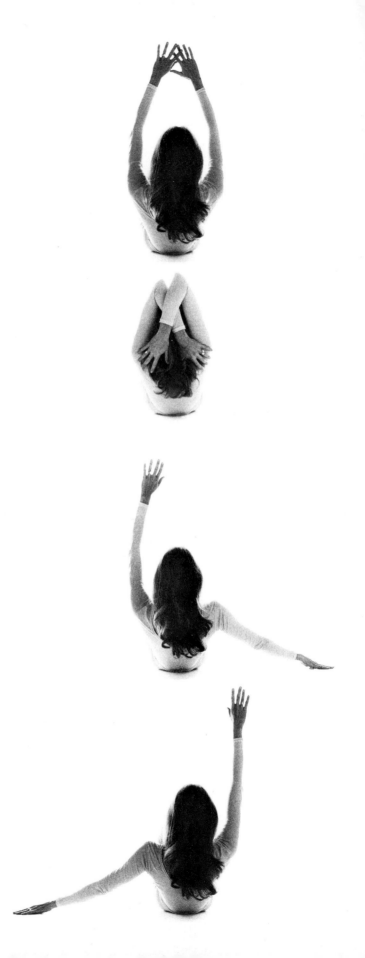

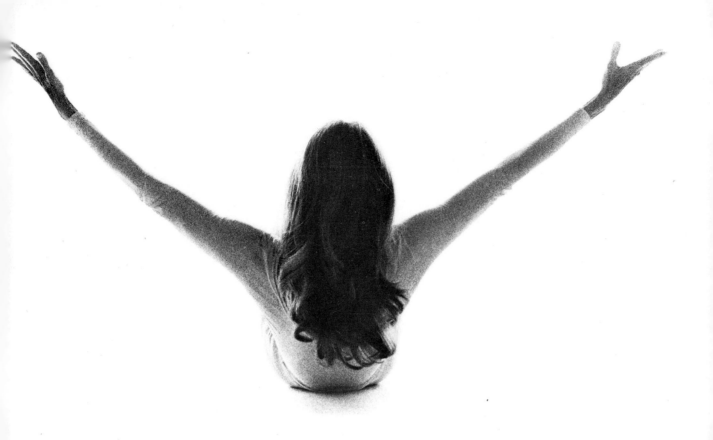

23 This stomach exercise is the most basic of all
the stomach exercises, but your legs do need
to be stretched so you can kick as high as
the picture on the opposite page. If you're
working on your stretches now and aren't
very stretched out yet, come back to this
exercise in a couple of weeks. To achieve
the same position as the last picture, you
need a good leg stretch. Even if you're
stretched enough for "the big walk" be sure
you have done all your warm-ups and
stretches before you try this movement.

*Keep your knees straight throughout this
entire exercise* and lie flat on your back.
Raise one leg as high as you can, aiming for
a 90° angle. The importance of the 90° angle
cannot be stressed enough. When the raised
leg is absolutely perpendicular to the floor,
your back will be flat on the floor. You
cannot arch your back in this position.

Lift your other leg a few inches off the
floor. Now raise your head and shoulders off
the floor. With both hands grasp the skyward
leg to "round the back." Keep the small of
your back in constant contact with the floor.
Let your hands go and, maintaining the
curved back, "walk" with both legs in wide
scissor strides, always keeping the lower leg
a few inches off the floor while the upper
leg is perpendicular to the floor. For the first
2 weeks grasp the back of the knee at each
high "kick" to make sure your back stays
rounded and doesn't straighten out or drop.
Later your stomach muscles will be strong
enough for you to kick and keep your back
rounded without the aid of your hands.

Beginners: try 6 strides.
Advanced: try 10–12 strides.

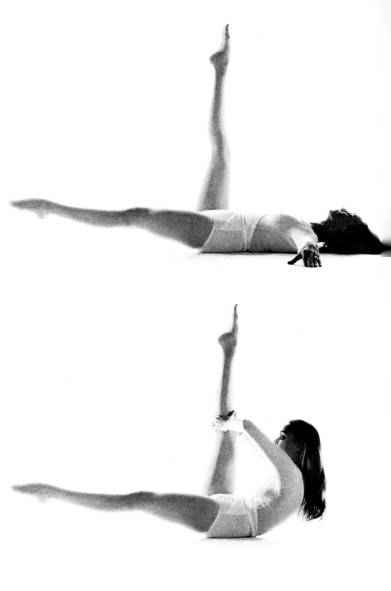

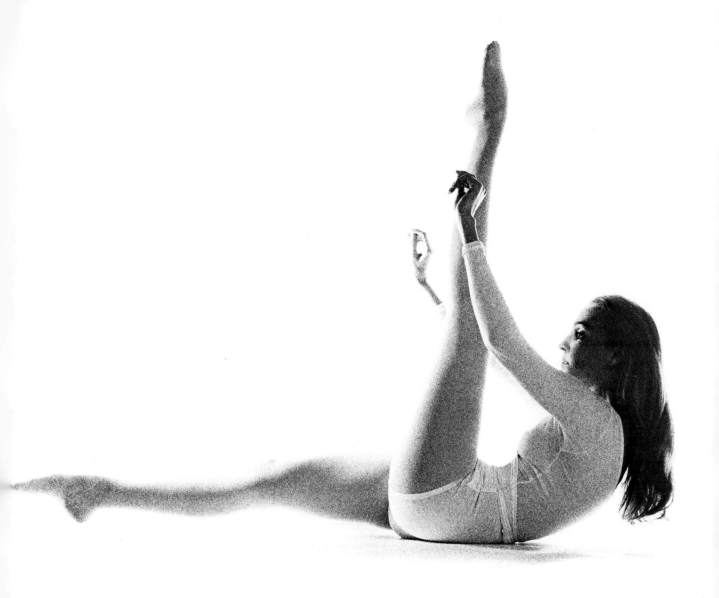

24 Any beginner can do this exercise. Lie on
your back with knees bent and stretch both
arms above your head. Arch your back very
strongly. Now flatten your back to the floor
pulling your stomach in. Feel as if you're
trying to pull your stomach muscles toward
your spine. Making sure the small of the back
is still touching the floor, slowly raise your
head, arms, and then your shoulders off the
floor. Hold for 5 seconds. A goal for this
exercise is to repeat these 4 steps 10 times.
Arch, flatten, raise and hold are the 4 steps.
It's soothing for aches in the lower back and
eases menstrual cramps by releasing tension
in the abdominal muscles. Many women tell
me they are going to have to miss class
because their cramps are so painful. Every
woman I have persuaded to do her stomach
exercises has thanked me and said the
cramps diminished and, in many cases,
disappeared.

Repeat 10 times holding for 5 seconds.

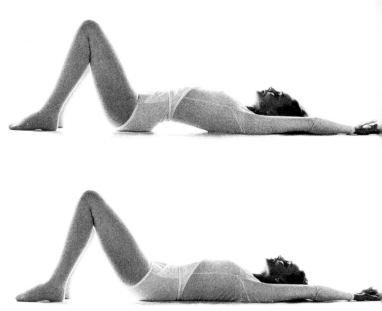

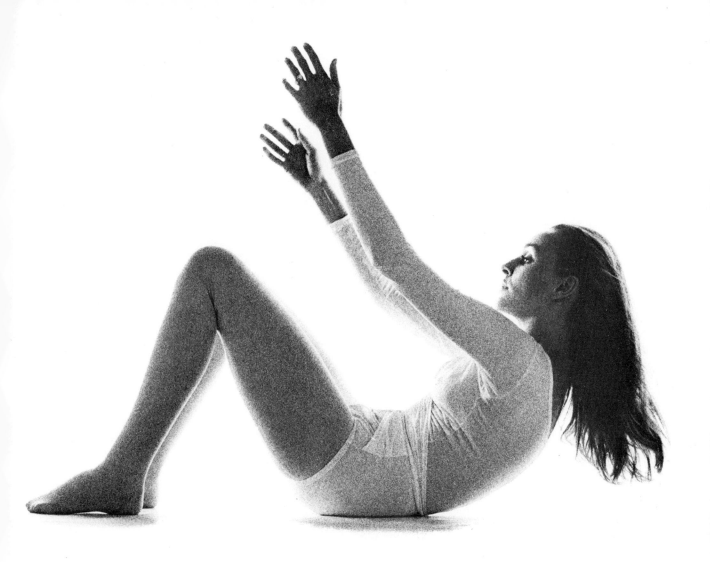

25 You don't need a bar to be able to do this
    exercise. You can use a wall instead. Position
    yourself as I have in the picture. Lie down
    facing the wall with your seat about 2 feet
    away. Rest your legs on the wall, pressing
    the bottoms of your feet against the wall.

    Raise your head and shoulders off the
    floor, letting your back come up round as
    you've learned in the previous exercises.
    Try to reach your feet with your fingertips.
    When the body starts to come back down to
    the floor, stop midway, which we'll define as
    the point at which the small of your back
    meets the floor. At this point grasp the
    outside of your legs and actually "round
    your back" by pulling on your legs. Let go
    of your hands, but be careful not to let your
    back drop down. Open your arms wide and
    try to reach back up and touch your toes.
    Slowly lower your body to the floor. The legs
    should be straight during this movement so
    you'll feel a stretch and a tightening in the
    entire length of your legs. But, primarily, this
    feat of touching your feet is achieved through
    your stomach muscles. In the beginning
    don't worry if you can't reach your feet. The
    upward movement alone will use your
    stomach muscles. You might call this
    exercise a sophisticated sit-up.

    Repeat 10 times.

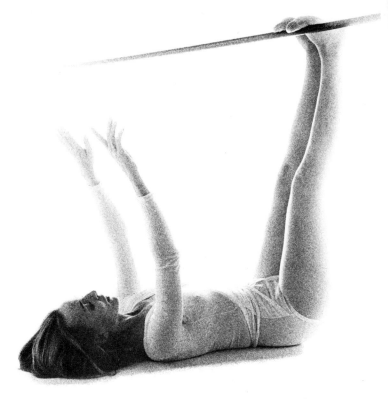

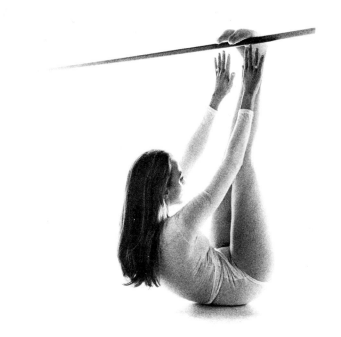

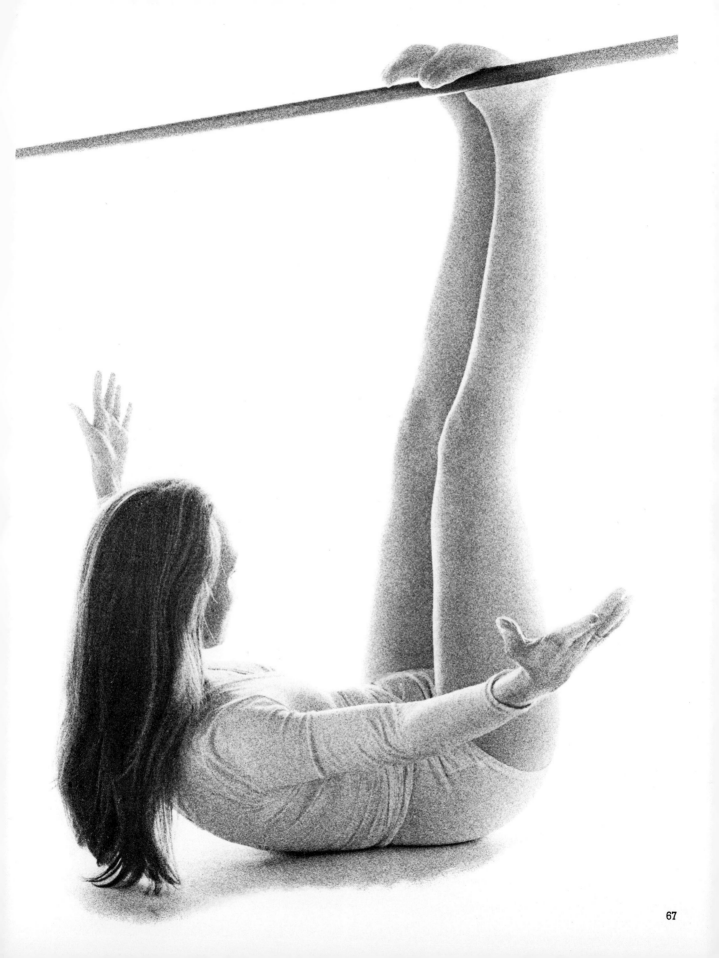

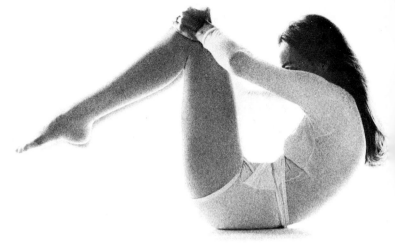

26 Warning : You must have very strong stomach muscles for this exercise.

These positions prepare the stomach for tasks as great as the half-moon position shown in the next exercise. Lie flat on your back, grasp your knees and "round your back," pulling your rounded back to your knees. Do not pull your knees to your chest. Follow the position of thighs and back in the 1st picture keeping the elbows open. You should feel your stomach muscles begin to work the moment you let go of your knees. Now! Let go and slowly stretch your legs and arms away from your body. To keep the back of the waist flat you may find that you can only stretch your legs up high, which is fine for the first few months. My legs are at a very low and advanced level in the picture, but it took me four months to reach this level! (If you feel your back starting to arch—pull your knees back to your chest.)

If you are able to stretch your legs out and keep the small of your back flat, try to hold that position for 10 seconds or more.

Still holding, slowly raise your arms behind your ears as far back as in the picture on the opposite page. It's tough! As you slowly raise and stretch your arms behind your head, you will create a greater tension on your stomach muscles.

Relax by pulling your knees back to your chest.

Repeat 2 times holding for 5 seconds.

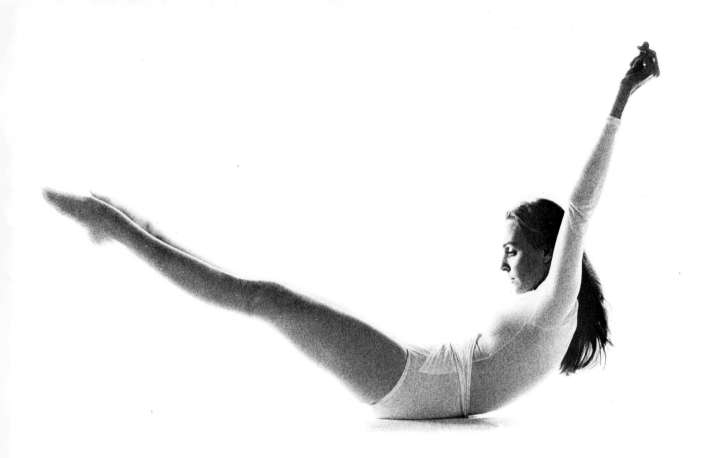

27 **Warning: If you are not a yogi, professional athlete or at a very advanced stage of body control and strength, do not attempt this exercise.**

As you can see in the picture, the back must be completely flat, the shoulders rounded, and the legs raised. The only thing holding my body in this position are hard-earned strong stomach muscles. Most exercise buffs will attempt this hold no matter what I warn, but unless you have very strong stomach muscles the small of the back will immediately arch and come off the floor. This is dangerous to your back because the back is then taking over the work of the stomach. Relax your body immediately if your back does arch. Lie flat on the floor pressing the small of your back into the floor. Imagine you're holding your stomach in as strongly as possible and all the layers of your stomach muscles are pulling in trying to touch your spine.

Next slightly round your shoulders and raise your legs a few inches off the floor. *Don't let your back arch.* The moment the back arches away from the floor, your stomach is no longer exercising. *Your lower back is exercising* and you don't want that, so stop. If your back remains flat with the legs and shoulders raised, hold to a count of 10.

Repeat 2 times. Hold to a count of 10.

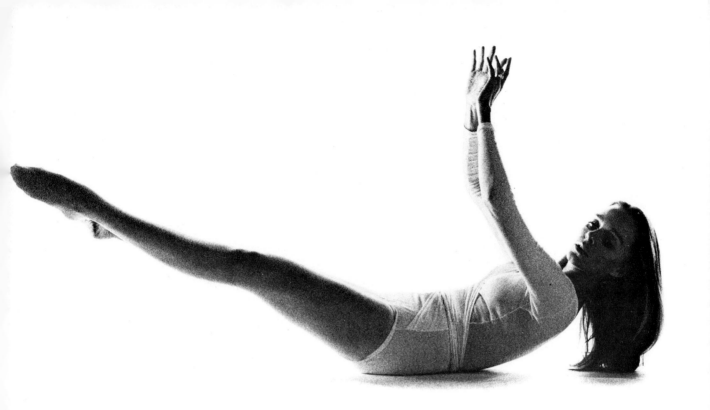

28 Pictures are much clearer than words in this exercise. Look at the pictures first and concentrate on the positions of the body and the stages of the exercise. Study the movement. Slowly look from the first picture all the way down the page and across to the last picture and then reverse—look from the last to the first. Now speed it up and you'll get the feel of this "torso swing."

Situate yourself in front of a fairly wide mirror. Kneel on your right knee with some padding underneath and stretch your left leg to the side. With your arms held high above your head, have a good stretch, feeling the stretch in your spine, waist, and stomach. Now for the movement: place your right hand on the floor and stretch your left hand well over your head. As you bring your arms outstretched in front of you to the floor, lower your bottom very close to your heel. Are you now in the same position as the bottom picture? From this position twist your torso to the left leg and grasp your left ankle. Stretch your right arm up high over your head. Reverse the entire movement.

When you have coordinated the movement, your body should be sweeping across the floor making a half circle. Reverse the movement and repeat the entire exercise 3 times. This movement is lovely to look at if performed rhythmically to some good music. When you are confident of the "swing," you'll be able to let your arms swing loosely.

Repeat 3 times.

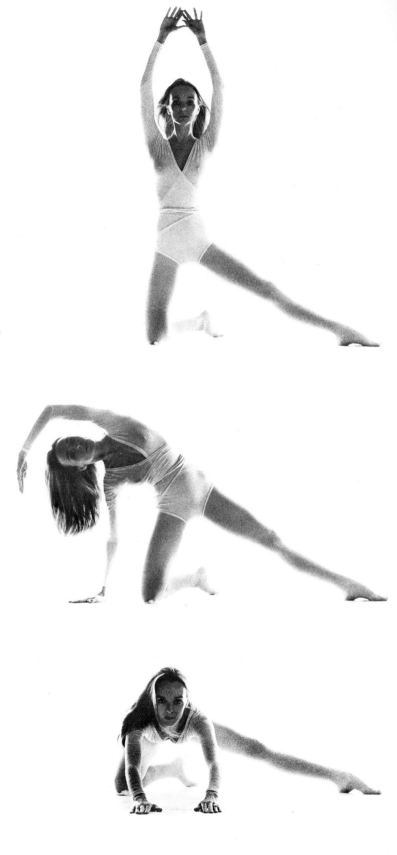

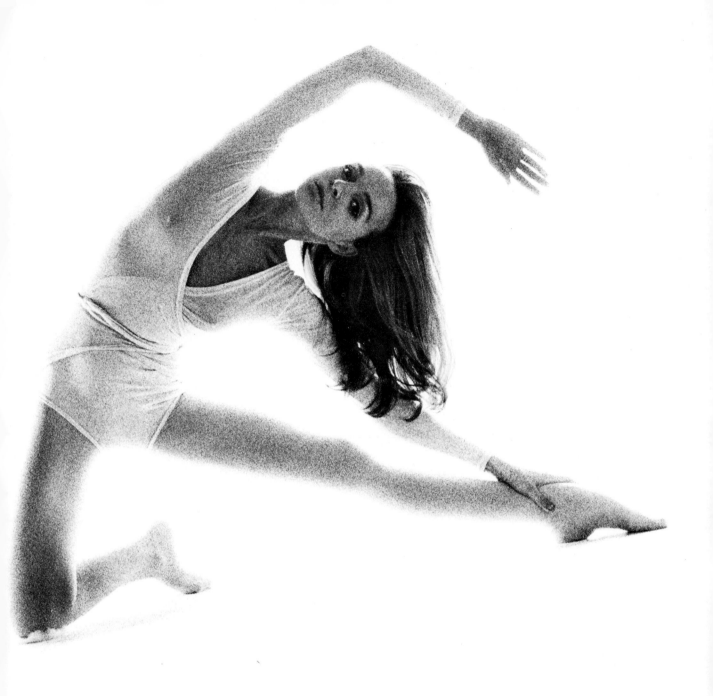

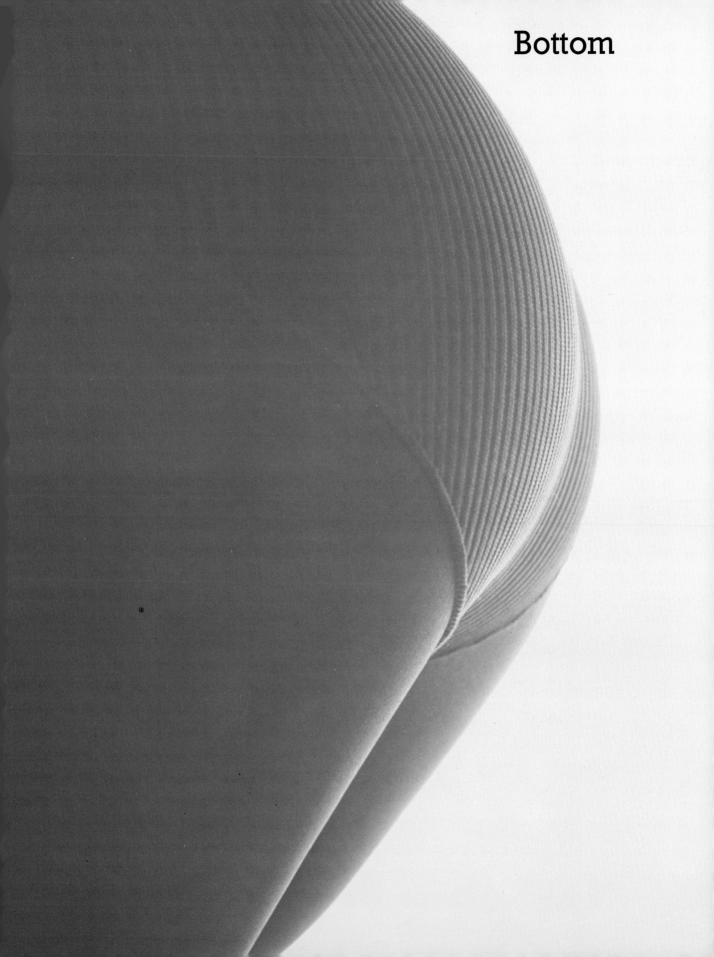

Bottom

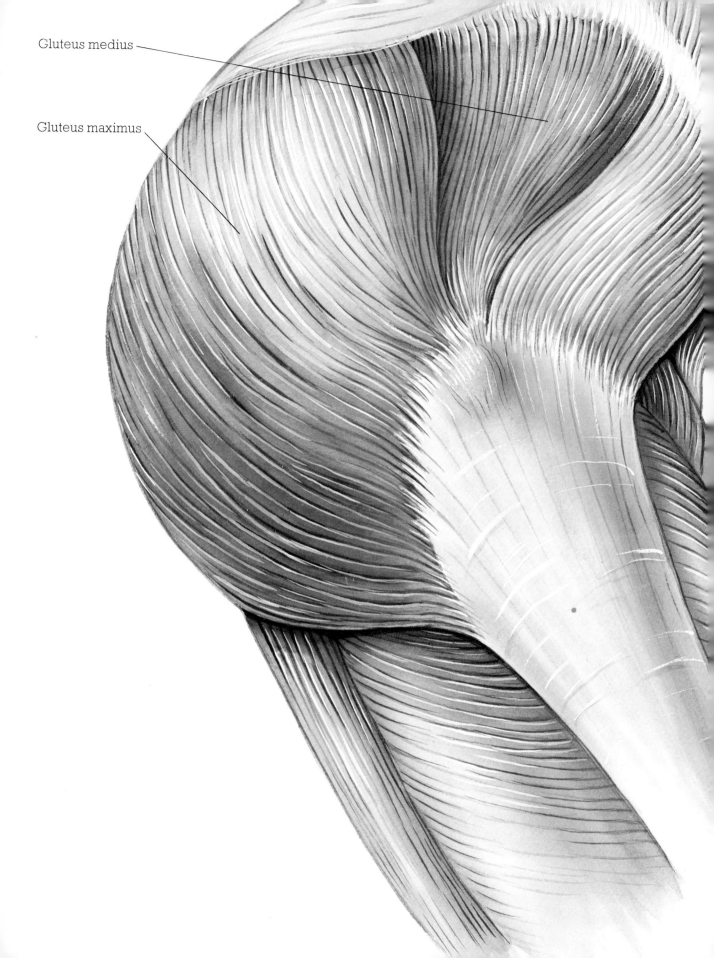

Gluteus medius

Gluteus maximus

Bottom

A ''hanging bottom'' is a frustrating condition but absolutely curable. It happens when the seat muscles don't get enough exercise. Women who sit all day should take special note of these exercises.

You can clearly see from the anatomical chart that the largest part of your seat is one muscle, the *gluteus maximus*. The muscle is in a perfect position to drop and make a bulge on your upper thigh. In order to firm that muscle, you must learn the correct position of the pelvis.

Once you learn that position and start to get the seat muscle working, you'll start to firm and pull up the seat—it's only one muscle!

In modern and classical ballet there are obvious differences in the position of the lower back and pelvis. Visualize a dancer on toe shoes with her arched back and seat sticking out. Compare that position with that of a modern dancer who has a tucked forward position of her pelvis and a fairly flat back. You want to learn how to *flatten your lower back and ''tuck'' your pelvis like the modern dancer*. In this section the word ''tuck'' is used constantly, because a ''tuck'' position places your hips at the correct angle so your seat muscle is used. Practice that tuck in front of a mirror. Try to control your pelvis. First stick your seat out, then thrust your pelvis forward. It's that forward thrust that you want to understand and be able to do: that is the ''tuck.''

If you have a ''hanging bottom,'' force yourself to do every exercise in this section. You cannot do these exercises enough. Your seat might get sore, but the pain should be welcome. Visualize a firm, well-shaped seat and the aches will be worth it!

Do the following exercises to music for 4 minutes.

29 Stand very straight, concentrating on the
pelvic area. "Tuck" your bottom under and
tilt your pelvis up. Raise your left leg inches
off the floor like the 2nd picture. The
position of the leg which is lifted behind is
important. The leg should not be directly to
your side or directly behind you. It should
be in between these two points. On a clock,
let's say, the leg would be pointing at
8 o'clock.

Keeping the "tucked" position of the
pelvis, raise your leg up and down about
5 inches off the ground. It is extremely important at this point that your outstretched leg is
perfectly straight. The movement of the
"tuck" and the stretch of the left leg causes
the hamstrings and *gluteus maximus* to go
into action. Try to do at least one nonstop
minute of this movement on each side to pull
up that problem seat or to make a nice seat
even better.

Holding your left leg in the correct position,
bend the knee slightly like the picture on
the opposite page and straighten completely.
Repeat the bend-straighten movement 10
times. You should feel a definite tightening
in your seat muscle. Change legs and repeat
10 times on your right side.

Spend 2 minutes for both exercises.

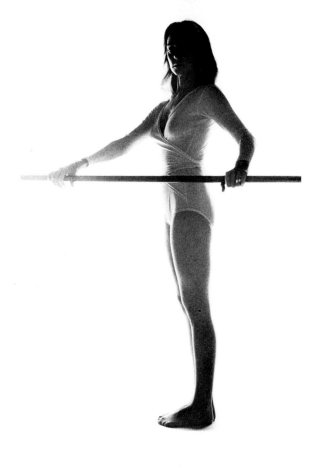

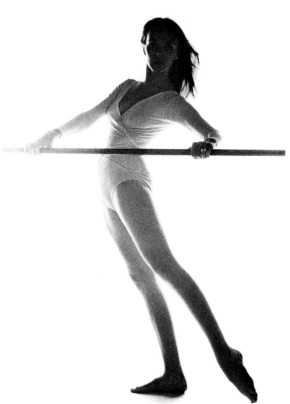

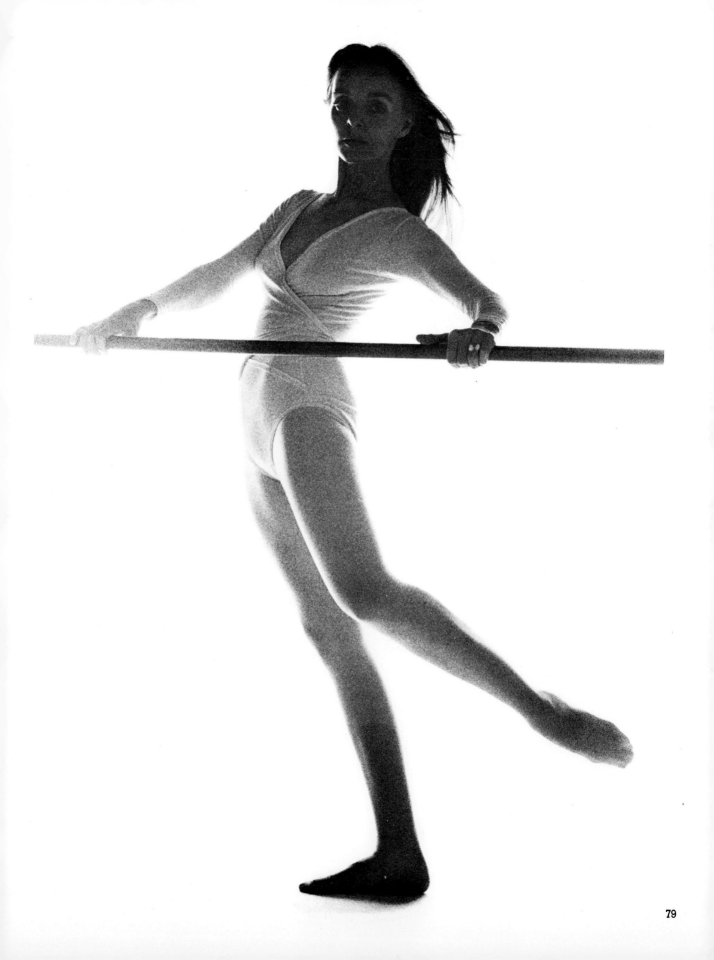

30 Kneel in front of a shoulder-high dresser and
grip firmly.

Press your pelvis flat against the dresser,
keeping your back very straight. You should
be trying to "tuck your pelvis" as has been
explained throughout the chapter.

Lift one knee keeping the knee bent as in
the large picture. Make small forward and
backward motions moving your knee several
inches in each direction, but keep the pelvis
"tucked" and flat against the dresser. Don't
let it pull away. Only your leg will move back
and forth.

Push the leg behind you, then bring it back
to the first position. This push tightens the
buttocks and pulls up that falling behind.

Twelve back-and-forth thrusts with each leg
is good for beginners or advanced.

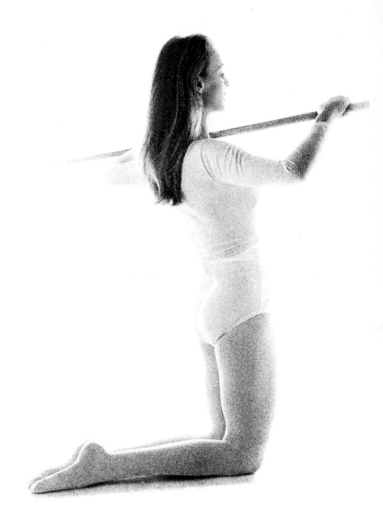

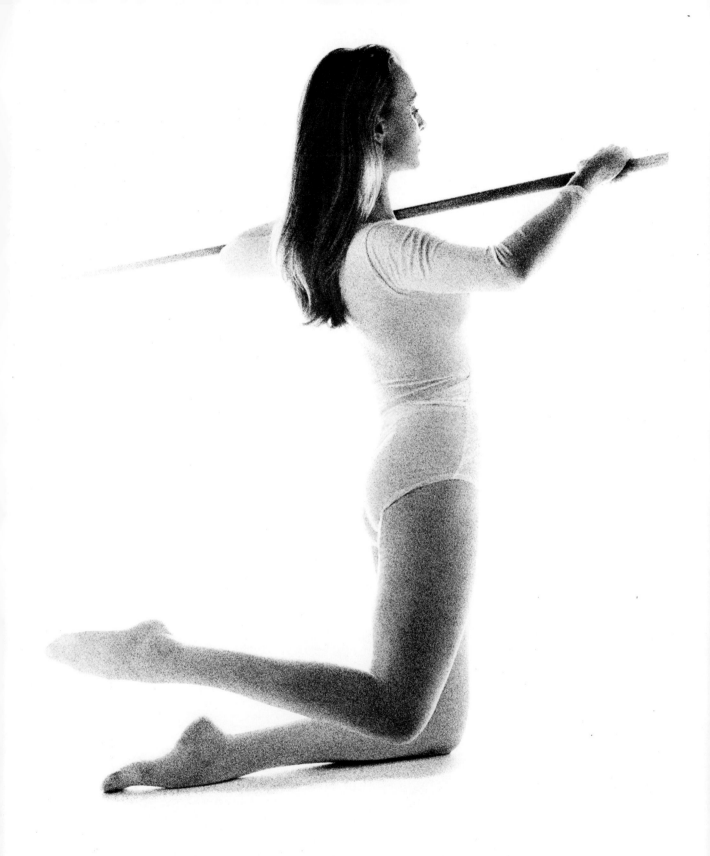

31 **If you feel any discomfort in your back when you try the exercises on this page, leave these out. It is possible that these exercises could aggravate back problems.**

These two exercises are reminiscent of the yoga position, the *locust pose*. If performed faithfully the seat muscles and hamstrings will become firmer and pull up higher.

Place a soft pillow under your pubic bone. Lie flat on the pillow with your arms and legs outstretched. Simultaneously lift your legs and arms as high as you can and hold this position to a count of 10. Lower your body. Relax.

Repeat entire exercise twice for beginners and 6 times for advanced.

A second variation: while *holding* the up position, bend your knees very slightly and straighten them, bend–straighten, bend–straighten, 3 or 4 times. When you bend your knees, you'll feel a slight relaxation of the seat muscle. When you straighten your legs, you'll feel a renewed tension and working of the muscle.

A third variation if the first two are uncomfortable: if you feel stress in your lower back, try a slightly different position to that in the picture. Keep your torso flat with your chin touching the floor. Now raise your legs as high as possible, *but* keep your knees bent.

Hold to a count of 10.

32 Keep the pillow under your pubic bone as in the exercise above.

It's only a matter of the formation of your lower back whether you should be doing this exercise or the one above. You'll soon realize which one is best for you once you try. Usually women with sway backs can only do the above exercise.

Start this exercise slowly. If you begin to feel any discomfort in your lower back, *stop* —you should not do this exercise but instead refer to the exercise above.

Lie flat on your stomach with your legs close together and lay your arms by your side. Slowly lift your legs and arms simultaneously and hold as high as possible to a count of 10.   Repeat twice.

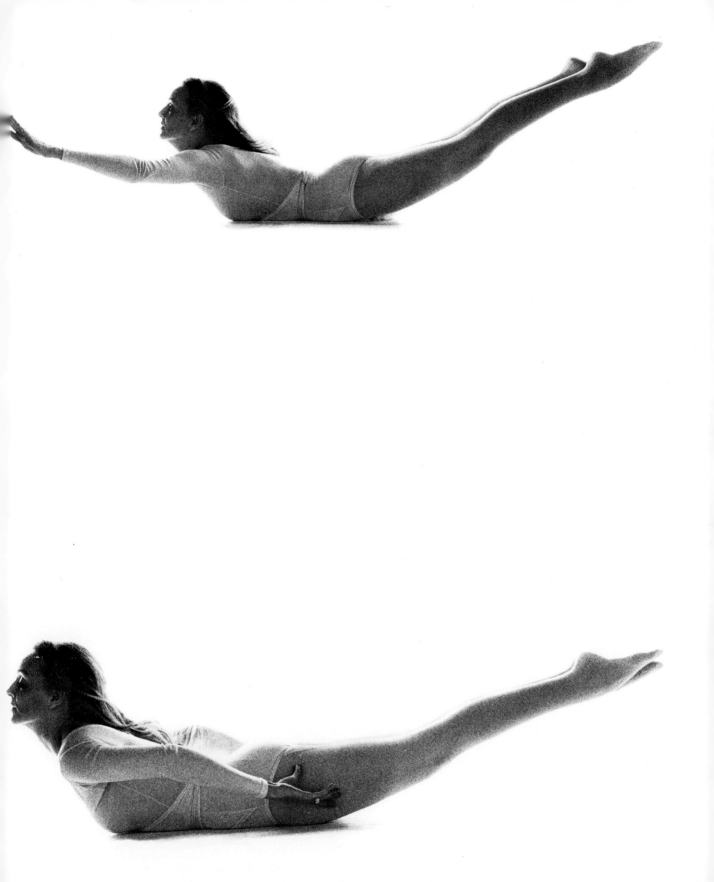

Sex

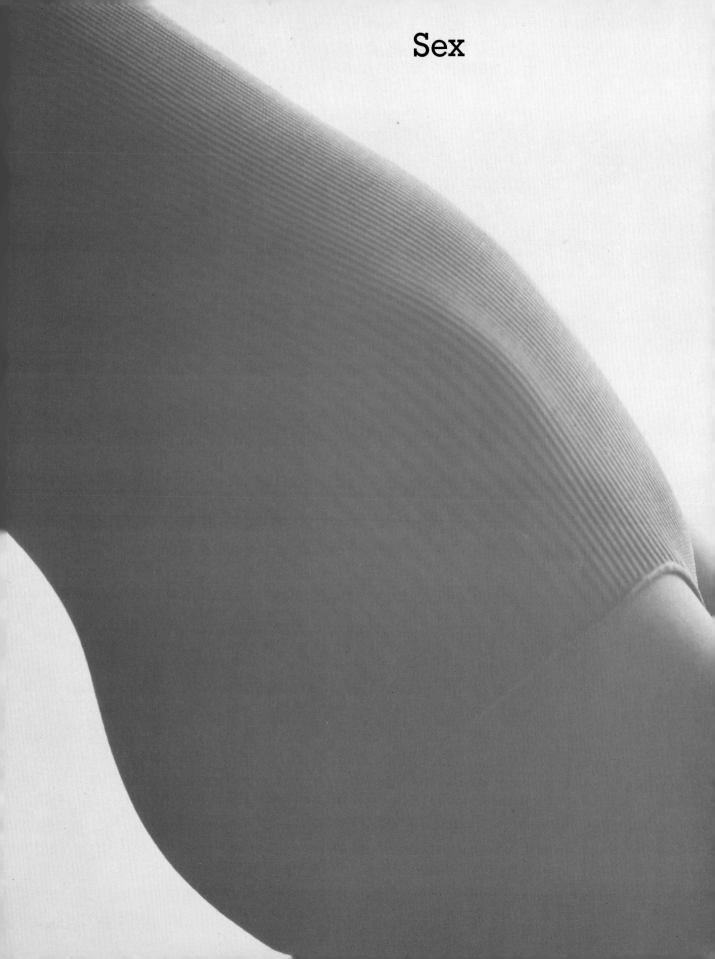

Sex

Everything about you is important in sex:
the tone of your muscles; the feel of your
skin; the movements of your body; and the
thoughts in your head. Your body should
free your mind. If your body is in great
shape—all firm, flexible, and controlled—
your mind need not be concerned. You'll be
free to relax completely and use your
energies to really experience sex. I want
your muscles to be alive and very aware. No
more "too tired" feelings. Well-exercised
muscles are sensuous and responsive.

If you're proud of your body and you feel
good, so will your partner. Whatever you
think of yourself is exactly how he will see
you.

All the exercises in this book are important
for sex, but your pelvic area is the source of
the movements and energy of your sex life.

Fluid and interesting pelvic movement
is best learned by dancing to fast or "rock"
music. Just relax and make your pelvis move
smoothly and loosely. You will find that the
pelvis moves independently of your torso.
While standing, put your hands on your
waist. Without moving above your waist,
move your pelvis back and forth. Remember
the "tuck" movement in the seat section.
Push the pelvis forward and back. The
exercise on the next page *really* shows that
movement. You'll need to exercise on a
carpet, in front of a mirror. Play music with
an exciting beat and start to get some
control of your pelvis.

Spend 3 minutes on these pelvic exercises.

33   I get reports from my clients that their hus-
bands have never seen them "exercise"
like this before. Pelvic exercises done on
your knees are fun if you keep the music loud
and clear. Once you position yourself cor-
rectly, the pelvis can be moved seductively,
coquettishly, or any way that inspires you.
There is so much grace to this movement,
and at the same time, you are firming your
thighs, bottom, and the backs of your legs.
(You especially firm the inner thighs if you
know just how to move your pelvis.)

   Turn on the music and kneel. Put your
hands on your hips or stretch them out to
your side, whichever feels more comfortable. Now move your pelvis as if you were
dancing to the beat, "hitting" first to the left
then to the right, or back and forth. You can
even make circles with your pelvis if you
really get control.

"Dance" for 2 or 3 minutes.

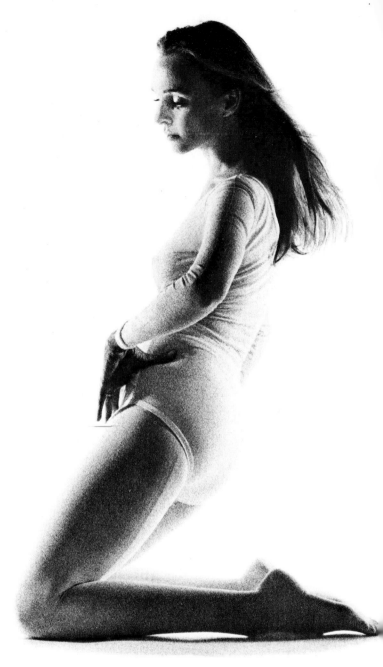

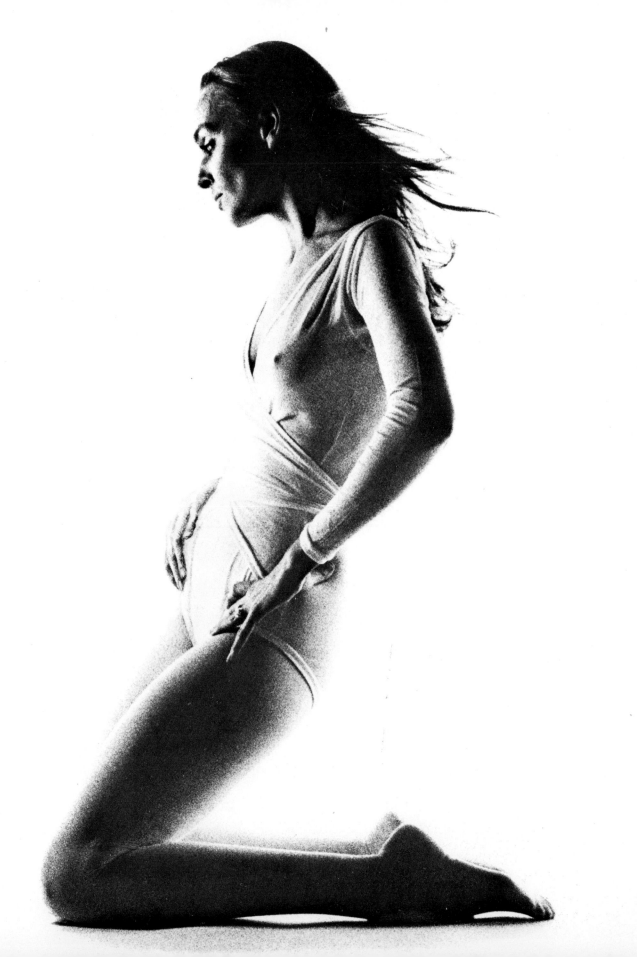

34 Before you begin this exercise study the
position of the pelvis in the 2nd and 3rd
pictures. This is an extremely small and
subtle movement, but you should feel it
immediately in your thigh and seat muscles.

Sit back on your feet in a kneeling position
with your knees together, and stretch your
arms high above your head. Raise your
bottom 2 inches off your feet. Tighten your
seat muscles and thrust your pelvis forward.
Stay in this "tilted pelvis" position for a count
of 10, keeping your bottom only 2 inches
from your feet. Now move your pelvis back
in a smooth snakey motion, slightly arching
your back.

Repeat the pelvis movement 5 times then
lower your seat once again to your heels.

You will feel a tightening in your inner and
upper thigh, and, as you can see in all three
pictures, the upper torso changes position
only slightly. This should be a slow, fluid
movement.

Beginners: repeat 3 times.
Advanced: repeat 10 times.

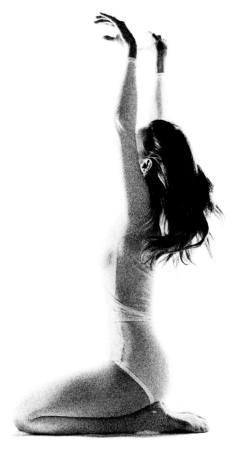

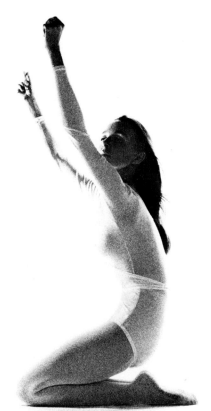

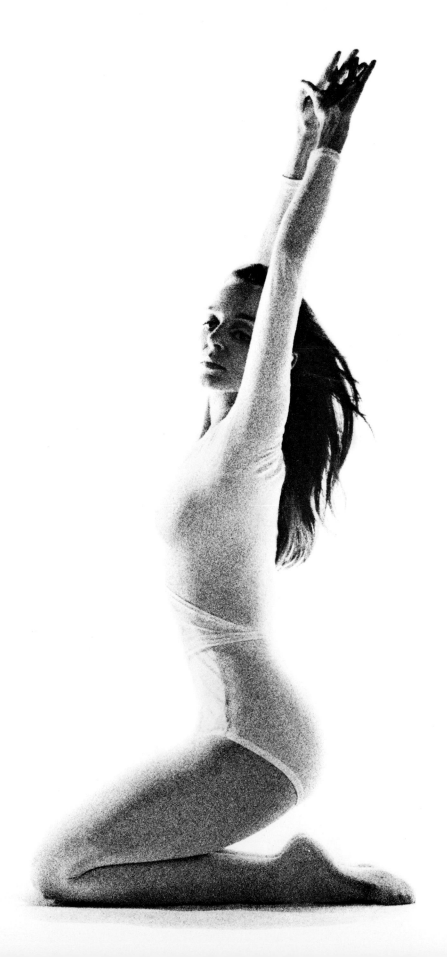

35   Although this exercise concentrates on the muscles of the thighs and seat, it is included in this section for the control, flexibility, and strength it gives to the entire pelvic area. If you bend your back, you will be taking the stress away from the legs and other muscles and transferring it to the back. In this book you are learning to use all of your body. By strengthening your thigh, seat and stomach muscles, any work load will be distributed. You will use your entire body and not just your back muscles.

  While kneeling, place your palms flat on your thighs and imitate perfect military posture with your feet and knees together. It is very important that your back be absolutely straight. Now, lower backward slowly using your thighs and a slight tightening of the buttocks. Keep your back straight throughout. When you have leaned back as far as you can, hold your body still. Raise your arms slowly above your head and hold for a slow count of 5. Now return to the upright position using your thigh muscles to pull yourself up. The object of this exercise is to lower your body as far as possible and eventually to be able to hold your body low to a count of 10. If you look back and forth between the 1st and 2nd pictures you will understand the movement better.

Lower your body and hold for 10 seconds.

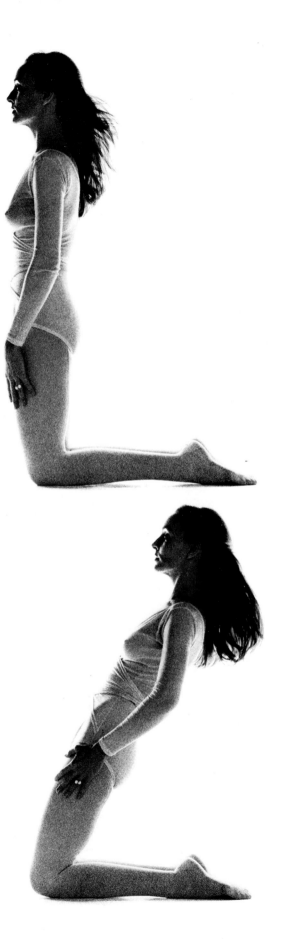

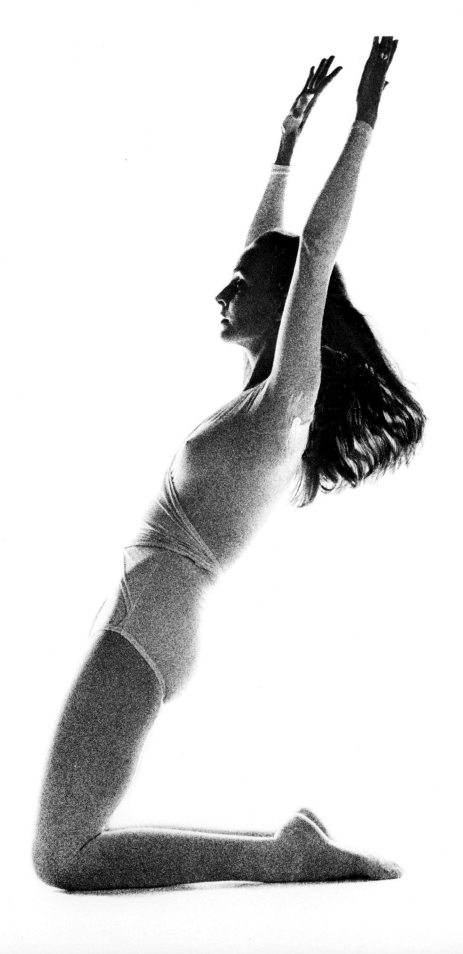

36 You can probably see that this next exercise is very similar to the preceding one, but it is a little easier. The knees are wider apart, so you'll be able to lower your body further than with your knees together.

Place your knees comfortably wide apart (12 inches) with your palms flat on your thighs. Thrust your pelvis forward or "tuck," as described in the introduction to the bottom exercises. When the knees are placed comfortably wide apart, there is less tension in the thigh muscles when your body leans back.

Remember the importance of a *very straight back* as explained in the previous exercise. Lower your body as low as you can without losing control of your straight back. All of the strength for this exercise comes from the thighs so you should feel the front of your thighs start to tense. When you've gone as far back as you have the strength to without letting your back bend, raise your arms above your head and try to hold your body at this angle. Hold for 10 seconds, then bring your body back to kneeling position. Ideally, you want to be able to lower your body as close to the floor as possible. *It is very advanced to lower even halfway to the floor. It took me a year to be strong enough* to lower all the way to the floor! Be satisfied with going a little farther back each time you do this exercise. Use a mirror to judge how much you are improving—the lower you go, the stronger and firmer your thighs will be.

Go as low as you can, hold for 10 seconds.

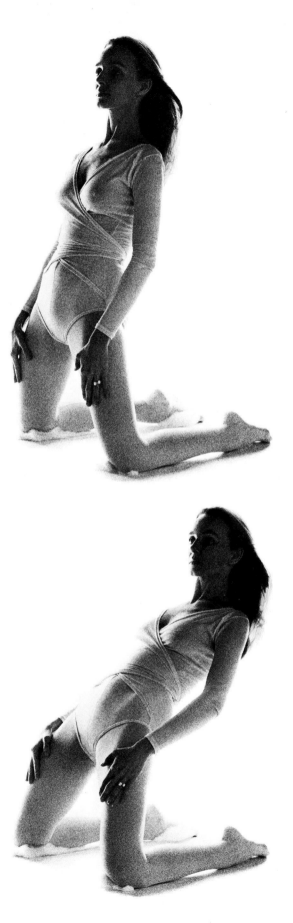

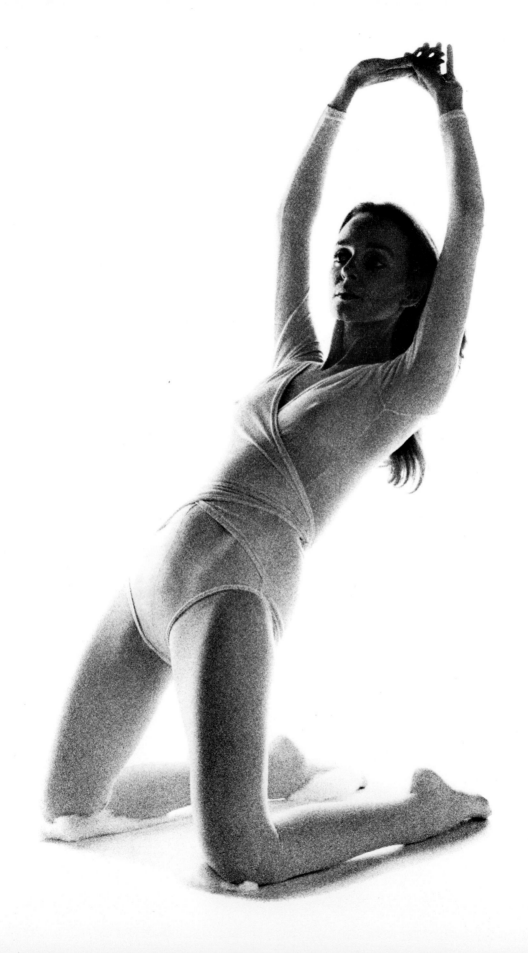

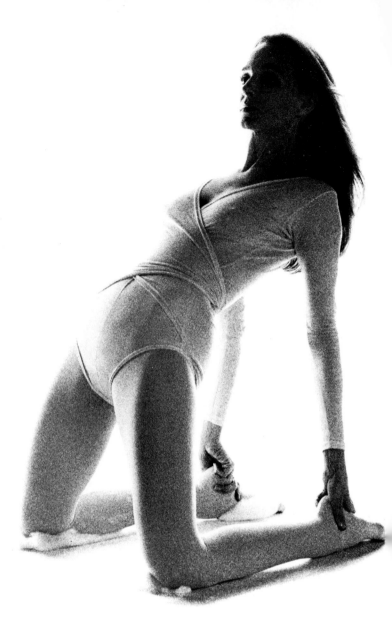

37 **This exercise is very advanced.**

Starting in the same position as in the previous exercise, lower your body far enough to touch your feet with your hands. Remember your back must be straight as you slowly lower it. If you are unable to touch your feet with your hands while holding your back straight, do the earlier exercises and work up to this more advanced position.

When your hands reach your feet, let go of your feet and raise your arms out wide. Don't change the position of your body. While you're holding still, count slowly to 5 and feel the thigh muscles tightening.

If you don't have any trouble with this exercise, start the exercise again and lower your body, placing your hands on the *floor* behind you. Tighten your thighs and raise your arms above your head. This is an advanced version of the exercise on these pages, so don't be discouraged if you can't do it for a few months. You've arrived at one of the most challenging parts of this section.

Lower, raise your arms, and hold for 10 seconds.

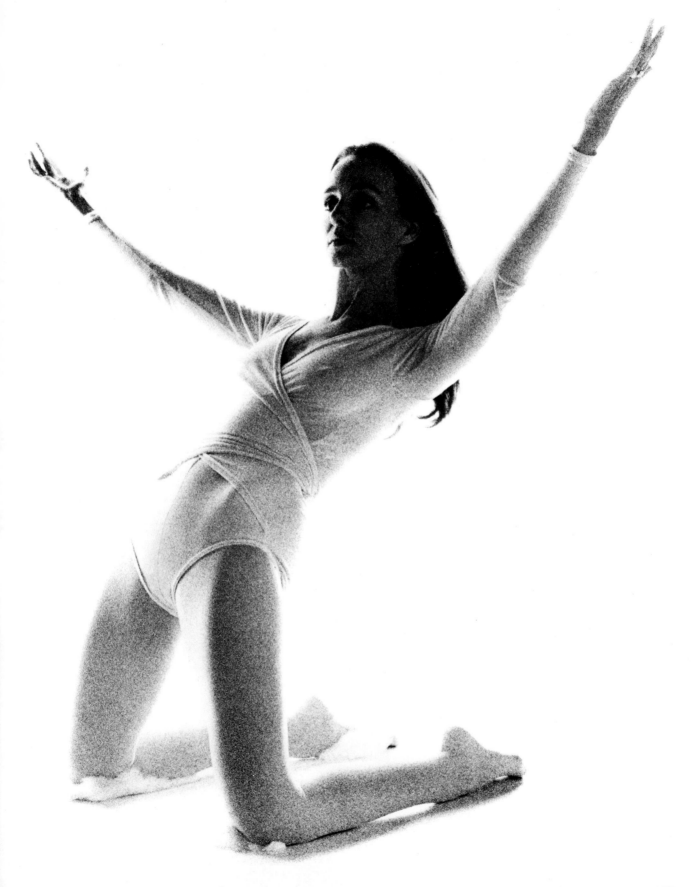

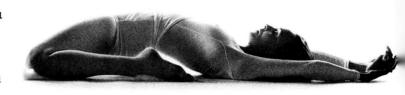

38 Do not even attempt this exercise unless you are very advanced, warmed up thoroughly, and can do all the other exercises easily.

This is the ultimate pose and movement for a well-conditioned body. I think even a yogi, professional athlete, or a strong ballet dancer would need to train for this exercise. *The crux of the movement is a straight back.* The crux of the first pose is an extremely limber body.

Open your knees wide in a kneeling position and slowly lie back on the floor. If you are not limber enough to get in this position, do not proceed any further. You might need to work on your stretches for months to get into this position.

If you've reached the first position successfully, stretch your arms above your head. *Using only your thigh muscles, and keeping your back perfectly straight,* pull your torso 1 foot off the floor and hold that position for *5 seconds.* Then raise your body slowly to a kneeling position. If you are able to use this degree of strength from your thighs, you have mastered this method!

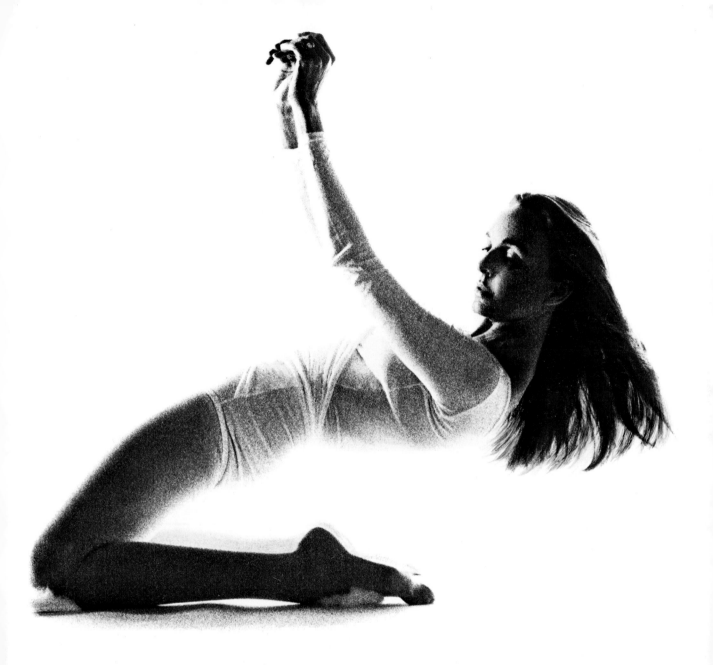

99

ABOUT THE AUTHOR

Lydia Bach grew up in Decatur, Illinois. After graduating from the University of Illinois, she worked for a year as a tax lobbyist, before going to Europe for several months.

For the next two years Ms. Bach lived in Asia and Africa, studying music, Oriental dance, Eastern philosophy, and eventually studying yoga in India. After working in Hong Kong and Bombay, Ms. Bach traveled for five months by land from Calcutta to Beirut. She then taught in Addis Ababa before going through Africa to Morocco, again by land.

In 1967 she returned to the United States and completed her graduate work in English literature while continuing to teach. After receiving her M.A. she spent a year traveling from Mexico to Tierra del Fuego, and while in South America, studied folklore and ancient civilization.

For the last four years Ms. Bach has lived in Madrid, Marbella and London; she is now living in Tokyo and New York.